'Fear and I go way back. Lil[...] fer from the wretchedness [...] thoughts, chronic uncertai[...] people have found freedom from fear, and I've found some of them helpful, but Rob's book has truly got under my skin. I love it that it's by a man. A self-confessed "man of little faith" who draws us into a narrative raw with experiences of deep hurt and trauma, yet completely abounding in hope. It's a book that has the power to plant seeds of hope in your heart so that, when the storms come, it's possible not to be afraid. Ultimately, it's a book about the One whom Rob has found in the darkest and bleakest of places, the One who remains once the book is finished. Read this book. It's strong, safe, good and true.'

Rachel Gardner, Director of National Work, Youthscape, author of *The Girl De-Construction Project: Wildness, wonder, and being a woman*

'Disarmingly honest, powerfully disruptive and reassuringly scriptural. Rob Merchant offers us all a rare and precious gift as he opens up his soul and the Bible in fresh and dynamic ways. Rob presents us with hard-won truth from the mine of deep and painful experience; humility and grace are redolent on every page. This book could help so many people.'

Dr Krish Kandiah, author of *God Is Stranger* and *The Greatest Secret*

The Revd Rob Merchant is Tutor and Director of St Mellitus College, Chelmsford. Upon leaving school Rob worked as a care worker supporting people with learning disabilities. Since ordination he has served in a number of different ministerial contexts and has worked in academic research. Rob's academic interests include ageing, mental health and trauma. He has spoken at events in the UK and overseas. His passion is to see people flourish in the ministry to which they are called, in whatever walk of life. Rob is married to Tamsin and they have two sons.

BROKEN BY FEAR, ANCHORED IN HOPE

Faithfulness in an age of anxiety

Rob Merchant

First published in Great Britain in 2020

Society for Promoting Christian Knowledge
36 Causton Street
London SW1P 4ST
www.spck.org.uk

Author's agent: The Piquant Agency, 183 Platt Lane, Manchester
M14 7FB, UK

British Library Cataloguing-in-Publication Data
A catalogue record for this book is available from the British Library

ISBN 978–0–281–08315–2
eBook ISBN 978–0–281–08316–9

Typeset by Manila Typesetting Company
First printed in Great Britain by Jellyfish Print Solutions
Subsequently digitally printed in Great Britain

eBook by Manila Typesetting Company

Produced on paper from sustainable forests

For Tamsin

Contents

Acknowledgements

Life has taught me to be a thankful man. It's taken time, but my life, am I thankful! However, this is one of the moments in life of 'public thankfulness' and the risk of missing out someone for whom you are genuinely thankful in a moment of 'thanking forgetfulness' is ever present, so please excuse some rather all-encompassing 'thankfulness'.

To all those who have journeyed with us – you know who you are – thank you for the utter beauty of your friendship that has lasted and lasted and lasted.

For my family, particularly my parents, who responded with deep sorrow and compassion when their 30-year-old son finally told them his story, thank you, for I have always known that you love me.

To my colleagues and many students at St Mellitus College, a place where we are each together being formed and conformed into the likeness of our Lord and Saviour Jesus Christ, thank you. To Pieter Kwant, a patient encourager of a writer who does (eventually) produce, thank you for enabling me to believe I could write again. To Tony Collins and the SPCK team, thank you for taking a risk and for shaping this text into what it is; whatever remaining flaws are mine and mine alone.

And finally, to my wife, my beautiful Tamsin, and my courageous boys. I give thanks to Jesus each day for the gift of love, hope and family that you are. I love you.

Introduction: The storm

I learnt to sail when I was ten. Each year my ordinary middle school took away a whole year group to a local authority sail-training centre located on the shore of an inland lake and enabled a group of ordinary children from ordinary homes to experience something extraordinary: the freedom to encounter that which cannot be controlled. Over the course of a week we sailed our little clinker-built boats around the lake, learning to work as a team and exploring how we could make our way across the water as we discovered how to respond to the competing demands of wind and water. That experience brought an unimaginable freedom; unimaginable to a ten-year-old mind and one that perhaps only now over 35 years later I'm beginning to comprehend.

My parents, noticing the slowly emerging confidence of their son, encouraged this newly found passion for wind and water, and a few years later my father took me on my first experience of coastal sailing on a 'big boat'. I say a 'big boat', it was a small day cruiser, but its mast, hull and little cabin seemed vast to a boy who had never encountered such a thing before, and I was scared. I didn't realize at the time I was scared; the racing surge of adrenaline with the promise of what was to happen caused my excitement to mask my fear, yet fear had taken hold and with each 'chink' of the wire upon the mast as the wind blew and the boat rocked against the jetty where it was moored, little by little my fear became more emboldened.

The day's sailing was to be a taster experience in coastal sailing off the Welsh Menai Straits, a beautiful part of Wales, the straits themselves separating the Isle of Anglesey from the Welsh mainland. The wind was blowing constantly but firmly through the straits and it promised to be a day of learning and excitement. Having prepared the boat, we motored out of the little harbour and into the straits, where we hoisted our sails for the day ahead, accompanied by an experienced sailing instructor in a small safety boat.

As we sailed towards the southern end of the straits, heading out into coastal waters, the wind picked up a little more and we made good progress. But the sky above us was darkening as clouds closed in, and the movement of the boat became more aggressive as the increasing force of the wind propelled us through the water, which was now beginning to surge and swell around us. Our helm quickly realized that the large genoa sail we had started out with needed to be urgently switched to a smaller jib sail to enable him to keep control of the bow of the boat, and my father made his way to the bow. Sitting astride the forestay, he hoisted down the large sail, which had now become stuck due to the force of the wind upon it. My father's courage in going forward was a startling image. I was fearful he would be thrown into the water as the boat surged ahead and thankful that he was willing to be afraid in order that the rest of us would be safe. As we headed towards the mouth of the straits, the call came from the sailing instructor to reef our sails because there was a risk of the wind increasing further as we headed out of the shelter of the straits. Reducing our sail area, checking our safety equipment and clipping harnesses to a safety wire, we were ready for what was ahead.

A force-6 wind strength is generally considered the safe maximum wind strength for inland sailors like myself. I was used to using my body to 'balance' the boat; tuck my feet under a toe strap and place as much of my body as possible out of the water in order to counteract the force of the wind against the boat's sail so as to keep the hull at its fastest point of movement through the water. It is an exhilarating experience, with your head at times skimming the surface of the water, the wind compelling you on, and the only thing preventing you from capsizing is the sheer determination not to be beaten by the unseen force you're battling through body and skill. Nothing had ever prepared me for the experience of when that unseen force is overwhelming in its violence.

My fear had by now safely overpowered my excitement and locked it up in the small cabin, where I longed to be so I could quietly weep out my fears, cover my head and hope like crazy it would all be over soon. My father was shouting encouragement to me, though I could not hear him over the sound of the wind, which was now, as we left the shelter of the straits, gusting storm force 10+. Never before in my short life as a dinghy sailor had I not been able to balance the boat, never before had I not been able to adjust my course or sail to spill the wind, running away from its force, and never before had I fully realized my utter vulnerability. As the wind struck the boat in violent gusts, which I had never before experienced, time and again the tiny big boat was laid flat against the surging water, my feet dangling out into space as the mast lay horizontal against the water, my body slamming against my harness as the water surged against the boat; and as the boat lay against the water I hoped against hope that it would come back up again. And as I hoped against hope the boat would right itself again, I longed that this could all just be over.

It's odd how our journey of life can be viewed through the lens of a story, the profundity of meaning only revealing itself in time as we are slowly reconciled to who we were and who we are becoming. Now as I think back to the Menai Straits and that 'big boat', I view it as a man not a child, through the lens of God's story, and find myself reminded of the utter fear that had taken hold of a group of disciples, some of them experienced sailors, as they found themselves caught between the force of the unseen wind and the ever-present surging waters; a story so significant for the early Church, that both Matthew and Luke recall the events in their Gospels as they recount the cry of the disciples, 'Lord, save us!' and the reply of Jesus, 'You of little faith, why are you so afraid?' (Matthew 8.23–27).

I am a man of little faith. I constantly stand amazed at the one who speaks into the storm and in a single command causes it to cease. I marvel at the fact that he journeys with me, vulnerable fragile me, just as he entrusted himself to a boat sailed by friends, and the womb of a young woman called to be his mother. But this I have discovered in my journey so far: each time the boat is laid flat against the water, in his grace and by his strength I am not overwhelmed. And as the boat rights itself against the storm, I once again glimpse the far horizon where only peace reigns.

Introduction

This book is not about great faith. It's not about triumph or accomplishment; there are many more interesting writers who can stir your soul to a boundless glorious action. No, this is a book written by a man of little faith who is slowly learning, on his journey home to Jesus, that when the storm of life surges with violence across our path it is possible, just possible, not to be afraid.

1

Fear

How on earth did I get here? That was the question on my mind as I waited for the pharmacist to sort out my painfully embarrassing prescription. Actually, that wasn't the big question, and it certainly wasn't the only question spinning around in my mind. The bigger questions were, 'Does the pharmacist look familiar?' 'Is there anybody here I recognize?' 'Am I far enough away from the church to make sure there is no possibility whatsoever that I might bump into anyone who might know me?' And the clincher, 'I'm sure that pharmacist is looking at me as though, as though, I'm weak . . .' Fear had taken hold of my heart; well, fear had taken hold of yet another part of my heart. Fear and I had become familiar friends over the years.

'Hi, Fear. How are you today?'

'I'm feeling great! Hey Rob, have you noticed that your heart rate is elevated?'

'No, not really.'

'Really? You've not noticed that you're a bit sweaty?'

'Well, now you come to mention it . . .'

'You know why, don't you?'

'Do I?'

'It's because you're going out for dinner.'

'Is it? Well, now you come to mention it I'm not feeling great. It's been busy today and, well, the thought of having to make small talk . . .'

'I know! You and small talk! It's emotionally exhausting; all that listening, all that empathizing, all that thinking of what to say next! And you know what?'

'What?'

'They've probably got extra guests coming they've not told you about . . .'

'*What!*'

'Yep, extra guests that you won't be expecting, and they will be sitting there . . . waiting . . . listening . . .'

'That's it. I'm not going!'

'Absolutely! Much better if you don't.'

'I'm, I'm *not* leaving the house this evening, and no one can make me!'

'Except for your wife.'

'Except for my . . .?'

'But she doesn't understand how you feel. She thinks you're weak.'

'How do you know?'

'I just do.'

'Well, I guess I am. But I'm going to be strong, I'm going to be strong and say *no*! No going out, no having to meet people, no no *no*! No one cares for me. No one looks out for me. No one loves me. I'm staying here where it is safe.'

'Well said.'

'Robert Ian Merchant, Robert Ian Merchant.' the call of the pharmacist repeating my name jolted me back to reality. Did he have to say my name out loud like that? Anyone could be listening! I needed the prescription I was waiting for. I had entered the cave. Fear had overpowered me.

It has always amazed me how a battle-hardened warrior like David ended up in the cave with this prayer captured in the words of Psalm 142 reverberating off the walls of his fear and loneliness:

> Listen to my cry,
>   for I am in desperate need;
> rescue me from those who pursue me,
>   for they are too strong for me.
> (Psalm 142.6).

What had driven an astonishingly successful, battle-hardened warrior who had earned the respect of his people into the darkness of a cave? David's story so far had been one of remarkable triumph. We are told that 'Whatever mission Saul sent him on, David was so successful that Saul gave him a high rank in the army' (1 Samuel 18.5). Yet when we meet David in the cave (1 Samuel 22.1; 24.3) we are left wondering what had happened to this great warrior of the battlefield. How had he come to be laid so low that he would declare, 'Listen to my cry, for I am in desperate need'? David's cry of Psalm 142 seems to echo off the walls of the cave into the darkness that surrounded him:

> Look and see, there is no one at my right hand;
>   no one is concerned for me.
> I have no refuge;
>   no one cares for my life.
> (Psalm 142.4)

For David, separation had bred loneliness, which had enabled fear to enter his life. We know that people cared for him: Jonathan the son of Saul risked his life to help David; David's own men followed him through various battles. Yet something had happened to lead David into a place of such darkness that as far as he was concerned he was alone; all alone without even his beloved YHWH present with him.

Back home with my newly dispensed prescription, I can still remember the utter misery I felt as I swallowed a green and yellow capsule containing something called Prozac. I had told myself that only weak people needed medication. I had told myself that faith would see me through. I had told myself that I was too strong for the sadness to overcome me. I had told myself all I needed to do was pull myself together. I had survived life. I had been successful. I was a leader. I had been president of my university Christian Union. I had been senior student of my theological college. I had degrees from two universities. I had succeeded where others thought I would fail. I had married an amazing woman. I had spoken at conferences. I was a trainee minister in a well-known church. I was fine. I was okay. I, I, I, I, I . . .

'I have no refuge; no one cares for my life' (Psalm 142.4). Deep in the cave, there is no warmth, no light, no comfort in the despair of utter self-consuming loneliness that denies hope and leaves you numb to the touch. We aren't told where David's cave was, and the reality is that our cave can be anywhere. I don't need to go to a mountainside, I can be sitting among a crowd, busy at work, busy winning people, but the cave is ever present, and I'm sitting in it.

'Set me free from my prison' (Psalm 142.7), cries David, but that takes breath, life and energy when the cave is an exhausting place to be. Perhaps that was the most shocking aspect; fear is exhausting. Fear exhausts us mentally, emotionally, physically and spiritually. Such was my own exhaustion that having collected my prescription, I fled. I went to a safe place where I slept, rested and wasn't asked difficult questions, I was simply accepted and loved in my broken state.

Of course, my wife and my friends had watched it happen. They'd had a ringside seat of my changing understanding of what I thought was normal; the steady reduction of my world so that all that was left was 'I'. That's the thing about depression: sitting in the cave, staring into the darkness, you're suddenly aware of how alone you are and, worse, you realize who you are left alone with. You are left with 'I', and all that does is disgust, because I am repellent. My repellent nature is such that I have managed to repel all that was good, so that I am alone. But in the ever-deepening pit of depression you miss how the loneliness occurred. You wonder why friends don't phone, email, drop by, take time. But it wasn't them who had lost contact with me, it was 'I'. I hadn't returned calls, I had ignored emails, I hadn't wanted to see people who wanted to come and stay. Because I was busy. I needed to focus. I was fine.

A few years earlier I had been reminded that one of the most common phrases Jesus uses is 'Do not be afraid'. Four profoundly beautiful and terrifying words. Beautiful because they tell me there is something other than fear. Terrifying because they caused me finally to acknowledge

I am afraid. But these words of the Saviour are not accusatory, they are not angry. In his voice I have nothing to fear, yet fear consumes me, and I hide deeper in my cave, longing to move further away from the gentle encouragement of love eternal.

Of course, we dress fear up these days with the more socially acceptable description of 'anxiety', which makes it sound rather like a doting great aunt rather than something lurking in the dark. One of the many boxes I have discovered I can tick is 'anxiety disorder', alongside 'post-traumatic stress disorder'. Fear loves labels, labels give it meaning, give it a mask to hide behind, because fear doesn't want you to know you are afraid in case you catch the words of the one who loves you floating into the cave on a breath of wind: 'Do not be afraid.' And it is a breath of wind, fleeting, momentary, brushing across your face and reminding you of the warmth of the day outside. It is too easy to reduce the Christian life to being either afraid or not afraid, as though you can be one or the other but not both. It is possible to be scared and excited at the same time, it is possible to experience hope and despair at the same time, it is possible to cry out to the heavens 'Why have you abandoned me?' and at the same time proclaim 'Yet you are God and I will praise you'. Read the Psalms – it's all there. The Christian life is not a life of polar opposites but of complexity, nuance and, above all, boundless grace poured out upon us by our God who loves and longs for us in the midst of our fear-ridden, hope-filled, nuanced complexity!

Some of us will have life stories in which trauma was either minimal or dealt with openly, bringing healing and restoration. For others, trauma will be deeply rooted and still felt each and every day. Human beings are a remarkable creation and our early life experiences shape the ways our brains form and develop when we are children. I am fortunate that following early trauma, my life changed in my later teenage years, when I became a Christian at the age of 16. Yet I cannot replace the events that shaped my story of life. My past continually pours into my present. That is always the shock about the past: we think we've left it behind, because it is 'past'. But that past has shaped us, has caused our brain to form structures that mean we are responsive to particular stimuli, that we find it difficult to manage the cortisol flooding through our system. The past, our past, is always present. The greatest task we face in life is to reconcile ourselves to the fact that the one thing we can never run away from is ourselves.

I'm not very good at asking for help. A therapist once described me as 'glacial'. In other words, I can maintain an icy calm exterior when all hell is breaking loose underneath. I have become rather well practised at my glacial, stoic calmness. 'No, I'm fine' is the reply to anyone who dares to ask if I need help. I mean . . . *me* need help? No, my role in life is to serve others, to be as useful as I can possibly be, to be as successful as I can, to be as in control as I can. Partly my response is founded in a British stoicism and deep sense of personal privacy (I do see the irony of that statement as I write this book), which finds fertile soil in my role as a minister in the Church of England. Called to serve, surely I am to lay down my life for the Church? I am to give my all no matter what, be prepared to make every sacrifice – okay, maybe I should add 'Messiah Complex' to my list of symptoms! But my outward glacial statement that shouts to the world 'I'm fine, thank you very much' hides a small boy still scared of the secrets he keeps while trying to be the man that he is.

Maintaining the outward appearance that everything is okay seems to be a fundamental requirement of modern life; the swan-like serenity that, while life may be a wild manic whirr of activity beneath the surface, what people see is calmness that exudes that there is nothing wrong, nothing whatsoever. It's a bit like the round-robin letters sent at Christmas, listing the various personal and family achievements during the past year: a mountain climbed, a marathon run, a house redecorated, a job secured, a new addition to the family. They are great to receive – I confess to having sent them – but they provide the serene outward appearance of success to the rest of the world when only those closest know the pain of a heart condition that meant the mountain nearly became a grave, the loss of a job leading to the loss of a home, the miscarriages before the long-desired birth. We can encounter the same experience with new forms of social networking. Look through your friend's updates on Facebook (if you're on Facebook) and see how many are truly honest in the moment. Of course, honesty is not what we actually want from people. We want everyone else to be okay because it means we can be okay – okay? The last thing you want to read on a friend's Facebook status is, 'Life is rubbish and God seems far from me, there is no one who can help me, and I am alone.' Yet that is what the psalmists did thousands of years ago: they expressed the honest condition of their heart, which was recorded and presented for millions of people to read through the millennia that followed. It is an astonishing gift to us today that speaks of the reality of living and following God in all his ways. I'm not suggesting that our round-robins, cards, Facebook statuses, tweets, blogs and so on suddenly take on psalmic proportions (now that *would* be depressing) but simply that we find ways to break the glacial exterior so that people can hear our desperate cry.

It is possible to maintain that serene calmness in the face of remarkable personal challenges. Therapists have suggested that I have experienced mental health challenges for most of my life, which are related to childhood trauma. This early trauma, which occurred outside of my family and which I kept secret until later life, had left me with a speech impediment that had a very negative effect on my self-confidence and meant I experienced a significant amount of bullying because children saw me as different. I was unable to say my name, unable to speak a sentence without finding myself knotted in a muscular angst as my mouth, vocal cords, tongue, my whole body felt as though it had come to a grinding halt. As I grew up, I would withdraw to my room, needing time on my own to restore my sense of personal calm. When I couldn't find the calm that I longed for in my inner self, then thoughts of ending my life would predominate. There have been times in my life when death has been deeply preferable to life, simply to experience respite from fear.

Set me free from my prison,
    that I may praise your name.

Then the righteous will gather about me
because of your goodness to me.
(Psalm 142.7)

The cave is a place of safety. Loneliness and desperation become very familiar friends in the emptiness of the cave. The darkness enfolds us, our voice the only sound to be heard. The safety of the cave is its familiarity. We learn what it is to survive the cave. We do not thrive in its solitude and silence, we merely manage to tread time and life, and exist. Change only comes when we are able to acknowledge that this place of familiar safety has become the prison that fear prevents us from leaving, fear of what awaits us outside of the cave: the presence of friends or partners who might show us love, the forgiveness of those we feel could never forgive our wretched lives, the bright shining glorious presence of a hope that never fails, never ends, never gives up on us even when we have given up on ourselves. Leaving the cave is painful. It is like walking on broken glass as love, warmth, hope, forgiveness, the simple brightness of day, are painful to the eye, the body, the soul that has grown used to the prison of the cave. I firmly believe that God is with us in the cave. Knowing Jesus means that the Spirit of God is deposited in our hearts as a promise of all that is to come. He is there with us – we cannot flee from his presence. We cannot escape him; David knew it was impossible to escape the presence of the God who loves us so much that he gave up his Son for us to rescue us from all that separates us from him. Yet can we praise God in the cave? David needed to be set free from the prison that held him for him to be able to praise YHWH.

Our stories of life shape who we are, and life is complicated.

2

Shame

I was recently leading an act of worship in which the psalm
set was Psalm 127, a beautiful declaration of Godly wisdom
and blessing: 'Unless the LORD builds the house, the builders
labour in vain.' It is a psalm that causes us to nod in agree-
ment. I mean, you can't exactly disagree with the gloriously
divine wisdom, 'Unless the LORD watches over the city,
the guards stand watch in vain.' It simply makes sense. Of
course we want the Lord to be the one who builds the household, of course we are going to long for the maker of heaven
and earth to keep watch over us, at all times and in all places.
I was reading out Psalm 127, declaring these wonderful
words to those assembled, nodding to myself at the wisdom
of Scripture, the glorious promises and reassurance offered
to us. But then I started to read the second half of Psalm 127:

> Children are a heritage from the LORD,
>   offspring a reward from him . . .
> Blessed is the man
>   whose quiver is full of them.
> They will not be put to shame.

And there was the rub, the breath-catching moment.

I'm infertile. In our marriage there are no 'offspring', no
'quiver' full of the children of my youth. In the time of the

psalmist my wife and I would have lived under the shadow of the question of why God hadn't blessed us, the question of what we had done to anger God in such a way, the question of who would keep our household safe in the frailty of our old age. And in a time when fertility tests didn't exist, it would most likely have been my wife who would have borne the greater question, the greater shame. My wife and I had tried for children for some time. We went for tests; my wife had an operation, which might 'solve' the problem. But it turned out my wife comes from fine genetic stock; the problem was me. It was interesting as a man to face the reality of infertility. At first I felt nothing, but the grief that was to come surprised me. Watching a television commercial with a baby, watching dads play with their children in a local park, tears would well up to be quickly blinked away. It was a sorrow that my wife and I shared, and a shame that I brushed away from all enquirers.

Yet an act of worship, 11 years after I had first been told of my infertility, caused my heart to unravel and shame to unsettle what I thought were still waters.

Shame is wretchedness within us. In a matter of seconds, I had gone from the glorious heights of God's promises to the shame of my condition. Yet in that moment I knew there was a choice. I could remain hidden in the wretchedness of my shame or I could speak about that of which I was ashamed and walk out of the hiddenness of shame into the presence of the love of the one who called me to follow him. That 'walking out' is an action I've repeated time and again as shame has attempted to cast its long shadow, causing a desire to hide and keep hidden that which I do not want others to know. But praise be to God! The light shines in the darkness, and the darkness did not overcome it.

'Where are you?' (Genesis 3.9) is the question that has echoed down the eons from the dawn of time itself, the question called out by the Creator whose creation was hiding in the garden; hidden, drawn into darkness, the long shadow of separation that would hang over humanity smothering hope, extinguishing the knowledge that had been spoken into being; the creation of humanity was and is the action of divine love. This covenant of divine love between the Creator and creation was broken in the wilfulness of humanity's choice to break the Father's covenant of creative love in an act of destructive faithlessness. It wasn't always that way: the Creator had looked upon creation and declared it to be good. However, the subtle voice of sin caught the attention of humanity, casting doubt and uncertainty in the craftiness of the serpent's hiss, 'Did God really say, "You must not eat from any tree in the garden"? . . . You will not certainly die . . .' There in the garden sin reveals its true horror, to open the eyes of humanity to knowing fully what is good and evil, and in that moment unleashes its lasting wound: shame, the place where love is turned to a pain so deep and utter that it causes us to push away that which comforts, hopes, forgives, serves, cares, because to be loved in such a way is to face the wound of shame.

'I know my transgressions, and my sin is always before me,' declared David in Psalm 51, lost in the shame of his murderous violence. 'Wash away all my iniquity and cleanse me from my sin.' The problem is, shame is sticky. It is as though no matter how much time we spend trying to wash it off, shame is a deep fracture in our existence tearing down into our very soul. Yet shame is not only a wound, a fracture tearing us from divine love. It not only clings to us; perhaps the greatest cruelty of shame is that it is repetitive. Shame layers itself through life as we are wounded by the effects of sin. In David's action towards and with Bathsheba, sin let rip envy, desire, lust, murder. A self-inflicted wound of the greatest folly, David's shame was the result of sin, sin that would take the life of Uriah, Bathsheba's husband, mar the life of Bathsheba and result in the death of a child; innocence stolen of life itself.

I know shame, I know its voice, its multi-layered effect permeating life, its chameleon-like ability to blend into parts of my life without my realizing. My infertility is just one element, for shame encountered me early in life in the abusive actions of others when I was a child. I was abused by two different people, both outside of my family. One abused me physically and emotionally, the other sexually, and it wasn't just once but again and again over a period of time, to the point that I spent a long period in my life when I thought what had happened to me was normal. The trauma of shame shaped my childhood brain. It made me vigilant of others who might harm me, suspicious of motives. It caused me to hide in the hiddenness of my mind, unable to sustain friendship. It made love seem strange and painful. Shame tore its fracture deep into my life, and the shame of it was that it gave cause for fear, anger, despair and unforgiveness that I poured out on to others. I wanted to crush those who had crushed me, utterly, totally, to completely wipe them out from any existence ever. Shame doesn't simply repeat within us, its repetition beats its rhythm out into those around us, those close to us, often without them realizing that it is the shame of another that is harming them.

How often I tried to wash sin and shame off of me, standing in a shower hoping beyond hope that as I watched the water drain away so would the dirt that seemed to stick to me. How often I would deny shame's existence, pretending that all was well, life was good, demonstrating to others my worth, my ability, all in the hope that they wouldn't see my worthlessness and uselessness. The effect of the trauma of abuse would physically affect my brain development, causing my mind to accommodate a world view distorted by shame; that what had happened to me was my fault, my lack of understanding, that I had been shown love, a special relationship that was always to be kept secret. In the battle with shame, survival becomes the key goal, surviving the pain of separation from love; a self-imposed exile from the self that means love becomes strange and unfamiliar.

My story of shame is not unique. Children and adults are abused again and again; sin and shame find themselves repeated every second of every day around the world. I truly have no understanding of how the Father can look upon his creation and see what it can do to itself. Yet this story of shame that we each encounter is a story that finds echo in the beginning.

There in the first garden, the Father walked in the cool of the day, calling out with a love that longed to see his beloved ones. In the shadows sat man and woman smothered by shame, broken, in the pit of their own despair, longing to flee from the presence of the one who breathed life into them. For the true sorrow of a forbidden fruit eaten was to know fully the utterness of shame and the separation from a love so passionate, a love so limitlessly expansive that that love was ready to span the limitless possibilities of eternity with a relentless desire to restore what was broken. The beauty of nakedness had become the shame of knowing nakedness, and from that shame poured denial, blame, anger, all the scars of the wound of shame that would become familiar to the lived experience of every man, woman and child.

The experience of shame occurs when we are caught out by something someone says, a reaction, a poor decision, a secret entrusted then shared, a behaviour we thought no one noticed now revealed. The immediacy of shame, so utter in our present, drives us into the shadows, to sit and hide and hope no one will see us, for we are made naked by sin, our shame exposed. Shame still regularly catches me out and amplifies my emotion. Early life trauma shapes our brains. It can cause the frontal lobe not to develop executive functioning skills, which can lead to difficulties like starting and completing tasks, problem-solving, concentrating, remembering information, regulating emotions, understanding different points of view. It has taken me years to acknowledge the impact of shame upon me.

In my various workplaces I've been known as someone who is highly skilled in some areas but not very good at administration. My brain finds it hard to handle starting and completing tasks. If the task isn't constantly in front of me, I completely forget its existence. Crises are brilliant for me; the demand of a specific task is utterly present, and I flourish. But the everyday stuff of administration in any job, I simply forget, or, more often, I think that I have completed the task when in reality I haven't. The number of times I've been surprised when someone has pointed out that the task I have been utterly confident of having completed *isn't* completed is, well, surprising. For years I've hidden this lack of ability. I've argued in job review meetings that I'm actually very skilled at administration, if only other people were better! I've minimized the importance of the administrative task and pointed at what I am good at. I've become frustrated at people's lack of understanding. And every time a manager has pointed out that I'm not very good at completing tasks and maybe I need some help, or 'training', I nod compliantly while desperately trying to hide the shame inside as I collapse in on myself, humiliated by my apparent stupidity that I can't even do the basic tasks in life. The shame I experience is of my trauma and the profound affect it has in my life, the way it has shaped my brain, the utter worthlessness I feel, and in my life I have worked hard to shield the shame of my trauma from others.

The 'Shield Against Shame' is a concept developed from work with children who have experienced profound trauma.[1] The shield acts as a mechanism to defend our shame, to deflect away anything that might reveal it to others. Through lying: 'I didn't do it!' Blame: 'It's his/her fault!' Minimizing: 'It wasn't that bad.' Rage: 'You always blame me! I'm rubbish.' Lies, blame, minimizing, rage – we can think of these as something new, yet shame is the ancient artefact of sin. Our recent scars are of a wound that goes far deeper than our immediate past or present. It is a wound whose depth goes deep to the first garden, the beginning of all things, and binds us to a struggle for the heart of humanity itself in which the serpent has continued to try and steal away the human heart from its Creator. Shame has captured the hearts and minds of many in our world. Created for relationship with the Creator, men and women still sit in the shadows unknowing.

Yet in the garden the Father's question, 'Where are you?' is not an accusation. For many years I had always heard the question expressed as anger – an angry Father, furious, shouting, expressing anger, instilling fear in the child who in turn struggles to hide deeper in the shadows, terrified in case he is found by the Father. I don't know where that fear came from. It wasn't a mirror of my own father, who has been a consistent calm voice. It was a visceral terror that was deeply engrained. My terror came from a deep small voice of the child who had desired protection, a protection that I wasn't able to give myself and for which I blamed myself.

When we have experienced trauma, we each have trigger signals that indicate our state of being. Therapy and reflection have enabled me to identify mine over the years. One of my signals is when I find myself late at night in a bedroom, before I'm able to go to sleep, having to check under the bed, in cupboards, behind doors, behind curtains, double and triple checking that the bedroom door is shut and locked, sometimes moving a cupboard or chest of drawers across the door to block it. I ensure windows are closed, because somewhere deep inside my mind I am terrified that there is someone in the room with me. It would be easy to spiritualize this experience, suggesting some form of demonic presence, and that what is needed is prayer. While I would agree we are in a spiritual battle daily with the one who would steal us away from the love of Jesus, our trauma signals can be exactly that – trauma signals.

I experienced my trauma signals recently on a trip to Rwanda, a remarkable country, people and context. It was a profound experience to be in a country that had gone through the utter trauma of genocide, and I spent time with survivors and perpetrators of that genocide to learn from them. However, each evening, having unwrapped my mosquito net and made my indoor bed in a tent of mosquito netting, I found myself on my hands and knees looking under the bed, opening cupboard doors, checking behind curtains, and double checking the door lock. The issue was not a spiritual terror, it was my past memory of trauma being triggered in the encounter of the trauma of others in a country affected by trauma. I didn't mention any of this to the students I was accompanying on the trip to Rwanda. My Shield Against Shame was busy minimizing and denying: 'How did you sleep?' 'Oh, I slept great, no problems at all.'

As I have studied theology over the years, I have reflected on the nature of God and the consistency of that nature. As I've been caught up in the wonder of the Incarnation, that God so loved the world he became flesh and set up his home among us, I've been moved to consider again what is the nature of God. John sums this up most simply in his letters. An older man who had had a lifetime to reflect on the person of Jesus and the nature of God, John had seen the storm calmed, the Saviour crucified and the eternal Son risen.

He had seen the growth and martyrdom of many who followed Jesus, and his vision had been filled to overflowing by the Holy Spirit. That man declared, 'God is love.'

Therefore, if God is love, and God's nature is consistent through all eternity, then the one who acted in extraordinary sacrificial divine love in redeeming humanity from the wound of sin and shame called out a question in the garden that was derived from love not anger. David described the extent of God's searching love in Psalm 139, when he asked, 'Where can I flee from your presence?' Yet it is only in recent years that I've come to understand David's question as not one of shame, driven by a desire to hide from the one who knows my shame, but as a declaration of utter surrender to a limitless, relentless love that pursues us across all eternity.

I decided a long time ago that I would not be someone who harboured the secrets of others. I was made to do that as a child, and in those secrets the shame of others formed and informed my own shame. No, the greater challenge has been not to harbour my own secrets, my own shame. To dare to answer the call of divine love, 'Where are you?' To emerge from the shadows and hiddenness of my shame, blinking in the sudden light of the Creator who is love. I still raise the Shield Against Shame, but I recognize it now, I understand its shape and curves, the way it has sought to defend me, but in doing so only separating and driving me deeper into the shadow. I've learnt to recognize the shield in others, to interpret its presence, and in the honesty of my shame encourage others to lay down the shield, that they too might emerge into the light.

3

Anger

In 2002, I was trying to complete a book and needed some time to concentrate and get everything finished to meet a contract deadline. My wife and I also both needed a holiday. My behaviour had been becoming stranger, and some friends of ours kindly offered us the use of a small cottage they had in Cornwall. You might have noticed the little 'complete a book' and 'holiday' paradox in the last two sentences. I hadn't. However, Tamsin had, and she gracefully endured me, who was only willing to offer a single-minded determination to complete his book, and my resulting refusal to engage in the holiday, with the argument that I had to meet a contract or I'd let other people down. Again, it's taken me a while to realize that what I was actually doing was saying to my ever-loving wife that she wasn't as important to me as what other people thought of me, so letting her down was okay! Don't worry, I know I can be a particularly unkind idiot.

The cottage was beautiful: a thatched roof, roses tumbling over the porch, an Aga in the kitchen and a lovely open garden surrounded by trees and shrubs, simply beautiful. It was the sort of place where you should really pinch yourself to ensure you really do know that you are there and it isn't a dream. A couple of days in and my writing ground to a halt. I was left with my own thoughts (not a healthy place for me), so I decided to go and walk around the garden.

I walked out into the garden, the bright summer's day casting areas of shadow and light. As I stopped and looked, a deep, deep hatred welled up inside me. A visceral anger that made me start to throw things, hit things and shout my hatred out, dominated my thoughts, words and actions. What was this anger directed at? I hated the beauty of the place. I hated the trees, the flowers, the summer's sun. I simply wanted to scream out my anger and rage at the sheer beauty of creation around me. I wouldn't recommend hitting a tree – it hurts – but I did. Raging at a flower does tend to make you look just a little deranged, but I did. Passionately hating and raging in the middle of a quaint English cottage garden is not particularly fulfilling, but I didn't know what else I could do. I hated what I saw, and it made me angry with an anger that emerged from deep inside my soul, with an intensity I'd never experienced before. This was no righteous anger; it was an anger whose roots were in fear and shame.

I've often looked back at this moment and wished I could liken the anger I experienced to the anger that Jesus felt at injustice, the clearing of the Temple, the frustration of those who lived outwardly the life of righteous faith but inwardly were as corrupt as the next person. The problem was that my anger was simply that – mine. It wasn't aimed at some noble cause or campaign. And apart from bulldozing our friend's garden into oblivion, which would have ended a friendship, I didn't know what else to do with it. An anger within me had awoken, and I was scared.

Anger is an exhausting emotion; it is difficult to sustain and when the adrenaline has finally peaked it leaves you empty as the anger lays bare the nothingness, the utter help-lessness of being nothing. I remember collapsing into sleep that evening, unable to persuade my body to do much else other than carry me to bed, and there I slept exhausted by my raging at the entirety of creation.

The intervening years were ones in which depression was diagnosed, a mood disorder suggested; counselling, psychotherapy, Cognitive Behavioural Therapy, various medications, and a great deal of prayer took place.

The psalms don't shy away from unleashed anger. Psalm 137 sees an exiled people so fired up with hatred that they desired the death of a generation of babies. So fierce was their anger that they could put their hate-fired desire in the final words of the psalm, 'Happy is the one who seizes your infants and dashes them against the rocks.' In Psalm 69, David's anger rises to the surface of his situation as he calls upon God:

Pour out your wrath on them;
    let your fierce anger overtake them . . .
Charge them with crime upon crime;
    do not let them share in your salvation.
May they be blotted out of the book of life
    and not be listed with the righteous.

As I read the psalms and feel the reality of the anger, I wonder again at the words of Jesus at the Sermon on the Mount as he reflects on the commandment, 'You shall not murder', and says, 'I tell you that anyone who is angry with a brother or sister will be subject to judgment' (Matthew 5.21, 22).

Anger leads us to places of hatred. But I was left confused. My anger was with creation, with the beauty of what I saw. It wasn't with people, so how could I respond?

In late 2010, I sat in a therapist's room and I looked out of the window. We were having a familiar conversation about my early trauma, the complications of abuse, the after-effect of a stammer and bullying that made me want to end my life, which I had tried to do when I was ten years old. A familiar conversation, in what was becoming a familiar place, looking out of a familiar window on to a scene that was suddenly unfamiliar. I'd looked out of the window many times before, but I hadn't noticed it before. It stood there, tall, proud, present. A symbol of longevity and beauty and everything I hated. The 'it' was a tree. It wasn't some magnificent oak, with a resplendent crown in full leaf. No. It was just a tree, an ordinary tree with ordinary leaves that I couldn't quite identify because it was on the edge of my vision in the far distance, innocent in its form and purpose, but it was there, and I hated it. I hated it with all my being, I wanted to swear at it, see it struck down, see it torn from the ground and laid bare for all to see, its roots sprawled in the air, victim to the violence of my anger.

And then I remembered. I remembered being a child surrounded by the beauty of trees, of primroses, of fern and bracken, of running water in gentle streams, and of hands touching and pressing, and deep within a childish fear not knowing or understanding what was happening or why the playful voice would not stop when I was afraid. And there all around me the trees had stood and watched, silently standing sentinel over my shame, the flowers and grasses crushed beneath me hadn't resisted or cried out. The beauty of that place had been witness to my shame and nothing and no one had cried out or stopped what happened. And I hated their beauty because they had not just stood silent once but, time after time, they'd watched inert, pathetic, disinterested in a child's shame. And in that moment in a familiar room, by a familiar window, I wept and finally I understood my question: Why had creation stood silent? Why did my rescuer not arrive? Why did God, Father, Son and Holy Spirit, allow a child to experience such shame and a man such brokenness?

Anger has roots that can run far and deep into our memory, becoming an emotion that can surge to the surface when our Shield Against Shame is triggered. Anger in my life was both suppressed and nurtured. Think back to the exiles of Psalm 137, sitting next to the rivers of Babylon, remembering the violence of their removal from the land, the enduring shame of their humiliation. These exiles were remembering stories of old. They handed down the visceral hatred of their victors to their children and their children's children. It was a hatred that would find expression in costly opposition to Roman occupation hundreds of years later, as hundreds and thousands would be massacred in their opposition to the oppressor. This would be an anger nurtured, suppressed and waiting for its moment, longing for rescue to come.

I remember sitting on a bench with my grandfather, looking out across the Bristol Channel on one of our regular dog walks. I told him about those who were bullying me, the humiliation they seemed to delight in putting me through on a daily basis, and I told him of my anger, my hatred of them. I didn't want to dash the heads of their children on the nearest rock, but I did explain to my grandfather how my life's intention was to become wealthy and successful in order to tear apart the life of each person who had harmed me. I would destroy them, I would destroy their families and their children, and ensure no one could ever harm or humiliate me again. My anger raged inside. I knew already that anger untempered, ill-directed, was a useless waste of emotion, but anger tempered, nurtured, feeding the fire of my hatred, that was anger that could accomplish my ends.

From the perspective of my life now I find my adolescent anger troubling. I wonder at who I might have become or what I might have done. What I do know is that anger consumes; it burns us up from the inside out and in doing so ignites sparks of hatred in the lives of others. Maybe my anger would have consumed me; maybe my anger would have consumed others. Anger dehumanizes, it turns its targets into objects. Anger has to do this, it has to objectivize in order to burn, or else we might discover that the object of our anger is a flawed human being, created in the image of God, just like us.

There are many places in the world where you can encounter that anger today. It is found in wars, in discrimination, in fear-gripped societies that reject the outsider, the different, the objectionable. I encountered its effects on a visit to Rwanda, a country in which almost one million people died in three months because of the anger-fuelled hatred of others. I learnt that over decades anger had been nurtured, suppressed, held in check, until it was ready to burst into the flames of hatred. In a nation in which tribal difference was little known before colonialization, Hutu children were taught from primary school that Tutsi children were not human, they were cockroaches deserving of death, a disease to be stamped out of the country. It seems astonishing that one group of children would be made to stand up in order to be humiliated and told they were not human. The shame of this was that it wasn't an isolated incident, but an intentional act by governments that wanted to slowly and carefully nurture a population to such anger and hatred that it could carry out the most hideous acts of violence against their fellow citizens.

I came face to face with this in a village community. Members of the community had gathered to meet us. They were representatives of a remarkable project that had been formed to enable people, who had been torn apart in violence, to rebuild lives and rebuild hope. As part of this programme, trauma therapy techniques were taught, and perpetrators and survivors of the Rwandan genocide worked side by side in sharing livestock to sustain and rebuild shattered families and communities.

During the meeting the various representatives stood up, introduced themselves and said a little about their experience of genocide and its aftermath. After several people had stood, a man stood up and explained that he was a survivor of genocide, that his family had lived in the village all their lives, that his father had been a village primary school teacher, and that his whole family, including his father, had been murdered, that he had only just escaped himself, and that the man who had murdered his father was in the room with us all. All of this had been said calmly, with care, grace and a measured pace of experience that left me bewildered when I realized that I was sitting in the same room as the murderer of this man's father. In fact, the room was a mix of perpetrator and survivor, but the reality of that hadn't hit me until that moment. This man, a survivor of the most brutal violence, whose family had been killed in the most anger-fuelled act of extreme hatred, was sitting in the same space as the person who had perpetrated those acts against him. Against his humanity. Against his very existence. And in doing so had left his life barren of family, of community, of hope – or so I thought.

It is remarkable how we can project our lives, our narrative, into the lives of others. We can be quite unaware of it taking place, but somehow my narrative of surviving abuse was caught up in this man's story of survival, and my narrative of anger and hatred was left bewildered by his calm, measured forgiveness.

The man sat down. Another man stood up, and the first words he said were, 'I am a perpetrator of genocide and I am the man who killed his father; his father had been my primary school teacher when I was a child, and I killed him.' The man explained that as a child he had been taught that his teacher's family were not human, that they should be exterminated, and that when genocide came, all that carefully nurtured anger burst into hate-fuelled violence. But then this man, this perpetrator of the most awful acts of violence, explained his life now. He explained he had been in prison for his acts, that he been released as part of a community forgiveness programme, that at first he was terrified that the community in which he had killed would kill him; and then he explained that he now shared a cow with the man whose father he had killed. He told us of the programme they were both part of, how they worked together in looking after the cow, and how their families had slowly learnt to trust one another again. My bewilderment level, which was already off the scale, suddenly shot into orbit. How could they do this, how could they not hate each other? How could they have found a way through the anger they felt? How? How? How?

I stumbled from that meeting room at the end of the community gathering. I stood back, watching the others who had travelled with me greet and thank all those who had shared their stories. The others in my group thanked both survivors and perpetrators with a genuine kindness and compassion born in learning from the lives of others. But in that moment my anger was sparking, and, in that moment, I felt the nudge of the Spirit to go and shake the hands of those who were the perpetrators, to thank them for their story, for their courage to share their story, and their permission to share their stories with others. And so I went, nervous, bewildered, and shook the hands of those whose hands had slaughtered men, women and children. As I shook their hands that day I was left with a question: Could I shake the hands of those who had perpetrated my abuse?

I know that I no longer desire harm for those who harmed me. Meeting Jesus cooled the heat of my anger. Today I don't burn with a rage of revenge that desires punishment to be exacted. But if I'm honest, if I'm truly honest, I don't know if I could sit in the same room as my abusers. I don't know how I could share a cow with them, let alone life! Yet this is my calling as a follower of Jesus, to forgive as I have been forgiven.

Perhaps what I have learnt is that the deep roots of anger are long-lasting. It is like a plant you chop down and think that when you have taken away the remains of its branches, when you have chopped it down to the base, then it is gone from your life, only for it to throw up fresh growth when and where you least expect it. Anger has deep roots, and the only way to deal with deep roots is to dig deep and dig them out – not only dig out the easy-to-find roots, but those that run far and long. If you've had to dig a persistent tree or plant out of your garden you'll know this is sweat-inducing, back-breaking work, but you'll know that if you don't commit to digging out the root, if you're not utterly intentional in seeking out all the places it has run, then it will spring back up, literally!

There are shortcuts. I've tried a few in my own life. You can chop the tree of anger down to the base and pour on poison to kill the root. The poison works its way through the root, rotting it in the ground. The problem is, you can't plant anything else in its place while the poison is at work because it will kill the new tree. Over the years I've used various poisons on my anger: shopping, pornography and being a workaholic are three that I've tried and found wanting. These poisons kill the anger, but they poison the ground from which new growth could come. No, the only way to root out anger is to dig, to dig throughout the journey of discipleship, to dig until the day I meet Jesus and am welcomed home, safe in the knowledge that the anger is no more.

4

Despair

Despair is a long-time companion of mine.

He tends to mope about the place, not quite sure what to do with himself, fidgeting, tense, a fog of intensity swirling around inside his head, though utterly unknowing of the purpose of that fog. Normally I ignore him, pass him by, deep in the business of my day, rushing from one place to another. I can look at him lost in the corner of the room, pity his rather pathetic excuse for an existence, and move on to the next activity.

But there are periods in my life when I can't rush about, when I don't have an excuse to ignore his existence. These periods are frustratingly called 'days off' and 'holidays'. Earlier in my working life I always avoided them. Days off could be resolved through a simple process of volunteering for the extra overtime; and holidays, well, holidays were my ten days serving as a youth leader on a children's camp. It came as rather a shock when my wife-to-be and I were discussing our future holiday plans to discover that apparently holidays were a time when you stop, rest, take time to do something different and relaxing. I thought this was utter nonsense at the time. A holiday! Stopping! Did my amazing fiancée have no idea that true Christian discipleship was to exhaust yourself beyond coping, making yourself ill, finally satisfied in the knowledge that in the utter tiredness and exhaustion you had somehow made God happy?

Made God happy? Who was I trying to kid! I was trying to make myself happy, or rather I was trying to avoid being faced with the sheer weight of unhappiness that marked my life. The problem is that when I stop, I am left with the reality of myself, all that I've been distracting myself from, and, in that moment, despair leaves its little lost corner and gives me a big embrace, whether I want it or not.

There have been some interesting moments in despair's embrace. Holidays in places of utter beauty that I've been unable to enter or see as despair constantly stands before me, consuming my view, demanding I give him my complete attention. A day off cleaning our home, only to collapse in a corner sobbing, tears streaming down my face, despairing at my utter inability to decide which direction to push the vacuum cleaner. It would be funny if it wasn't so utterly foul. The embrace of despair is soul-consuming; in its big ugly embrace despair sucks out hope. It is the ultimate suction machine: every last little bit of hope, joy, love is sucked out of you into the great vacuum bag of despair. But don't worry! Despair is a generous giver! It doesn't suck out everything and leave you with nothing. No! In its generosity despair moves in. Despair is like the ultimate cuckoo. Having kicked out everything good it settles into your life and makes itself nice and comfortable.

I first encountered despair as a child. Aged ten I was at a school where I found myself continuously bullied. Each and every day was a day of rejection, name-calling, isolation and being hit by others. My earlier experiences of

physical and emotional abuse meant that school environ-
ments were places of fear for me, as one of my abusers had
been a teacher who enjoyed making me afraid. If I made a
spelling mistake, I would be told to stand up so the class
could laugh at me, and told to stand in the corner for being
stupid. If I needed the toilet I wouldn't be permitted to go,
so I would wet or soil myself, and the action of being made
to stand up and be laughed at would begin all over again.
Standing at the side of the outdoor school swimming pool, I
would be the child the teacher would push into the pool,
struggling to keep my head above water as I was unable to
swim, only to be pulled out by an older child. Then the ritual
of laughter and humiliation for the stupid boy who couldn't
swim would begin again. Finally this daily ritual of humiliation left me with the ultimate evidence of my humiliation:
a speech impediment that meant I couldn't say my name
and that triggered a blocking stammer whenever I was anxious. Despair had moved in from an early age for me and by
the age of ten I was tired of despair's presence in my life, so
I decided that the best option, the only option, was to die.

Bullying is pernicious. It slowly strips away your dignity,
belittling your existence. My family lived in the countryside
and in order to get to school I had to catch a bus. 'M-M-
M-M-Merchant . . .' 'What's your name M-M-M-M-M-
Merchant?' The bullying and laughter would start as soon
as the door of the bus opened, 'Can't say your name can
you R-R-R-R-R-Robert M-M-M-M-M-Merchant?' The
children who delighted in making life miserable had no
idea of my story. They didn't know that the reason for my
stammer was my being sexually, physically and emotionally

abused by two different people over a period of time. They didn't know about the trauma of watching my sister be viciously attacked by a dog, seeing her flung about like a doll as I screamed at the dog to stop, only for the dog to drop my sister to the ground and come after me, her blood visible in its mouth. All they saw, and heard, was a boy who was different from them.

Poor mental health can make us a stranger to others. Your behaviour and words can become erratic, your decision-making appears out of the ordinary, your ability to sustain relationships is impaired. I wonder how often, when we meet people who are expressing deep and lasting despair, whose outward appearance and behaviour are strange to us, are we able to look beyond and take time to hear the person's story? To learn what has happened to bring that person to a place of brokenness? To hear someone's story is to hear the deepest anguished cry of their heart, their despair in all its desperation, and simply sit alongside and listen.

Context is everything. The depth of pain expressed in Psalm 137 is extraordinary because the context of the psalm is extraordinary. Imagine being taken away from your home, from all that is familiar, from the land that has sustained you, from the land that God had promised your forefathers, and now sitting as a prisoner regretting every moment of your existence and the past of your people. Psalm 137 is about the lived experience of pain and a reminder that despair can fire hatred in a furnace that would desire the deaths of a generation of children in order to end the pain of those in despair. The theologian Walter Brueggemann writes: 'It is not for us to "justify" such a prayer in the Bible

. . . it is not one of the noble moments of the Bible, but it is there.'[2] The psalm provides us with a historical snapshot of a people in despair, and tears away all pretence to reveal the open wound that can lie at the heart of a people. Despair festers, it poisons every area of life it touches, until it has spread and taken hold, utterly, completely, blocking out all memory of God, all knowledge of his wondrous presence.

Despair can hold us prisoner as our soul rages at the world and its cruelty to us. It can cause us to harm those who try to comfort us, because we consider ourselves alone and unwanted. It is astonishing in those moments the harm we can do to those who love us. I very occasionally speak about my experience in conference settings – only occasionally, because it is always costly, because I am talking about the reality of my life. At one conference I was asked, as a person with a long-term mental health condition, what was the main thing I needed from those around me, those who love me. The answer was simple: forgiveness. I need to know that I will be forgiven, that I am forgiven, for the darkness of my despair can cause me to harm those who show me the greatest love and compassion, because the strength of their love hurts. It is physically, emotionally and spiritually painful.

To be in relationship with me is costly. My ten-year-old self reached a point of such despair with bullying, with the trauma of living, that I tried to shoot myself with my father's shotgun. I knew where he kept the gun, I'd seen a shotgun loaded, prepared and fired, and I'd figured out how to complete my suicide. I also knew why I wanted to die: I was tired of the despair, the never-ending grinding despair of living. I was unable to complete my suicide because my father was a wise man, and kept his shotgun cartridges separately from the shotgun in a place I couldn't find, and just as I was contemplating which room I'd need to tear apart to find the cartridges, one of my parents returned. If you'd met me as a ten-year-old you would have met an ordinary boy. I went out, I worked to earn pocket money, you'd have no idea what life was like inside of me. Abuse had taught me to remain silent, to shut down all emotion, not to reveal weakness or fear, and certainly not to tell you what I really thought. A desire to end my life through suicide has meant that suicidal ideation has been part of my journey.

To be in relationship with me is costly. There have been times when my wife has had to sit and hear my deepest despair. To hear me speak of my desire to die and on one occasion to listen to me explaining how I'd used my internet search engine to find the most effective way to tie a noose so I could hang myself. To receive a telephone call from me asking her to pray because the desire to end my life was at that moment overwhelming me. My despair has never been turned outwards towards others; my hatred has always been of myself. People think the absence of hope is hopelessness, but it isn't. The absence of hope is despair.

Despair manifests itself in episodic depression in my life. Prayer and therapy have lessened the effect of despair over the years. Thoughts of suicide have been absent for a long time now, and my wife and I have both learnt how to spot despair when it's wandered from its corner to embrace me. We've discovered that in my life despair loves humiliation that stirs up past fear, and open communication is a vital tool in recognizing despair and the inevitable onset of depression.

Depression turns a person in on him- or herself, stealing character, bringing exile from all that was once familiar and opening the way to despair. Someone once described depression to me as a 'thief'. The illness steals away your sense of identity, connectivity to others, self-worth, community, hope. But you only realize the crime that has taken place after the event, when it is all too late to prevent. That person, a GP, was also the first person to tell me honestly that there was something very wrong with me and that I needed to go to my own GP and ask for help. Depression steals you away from the land and community you once knew, without you ever realizing that you had left. You wake one day to find yourself sitting in an unfamiliar land, wondering how you got there and despairing that you may never return home. You hold a vague memory of how life once was, but you struggle to remember.

The writer of Psalm 137 asks, 'How can we sing the songs of the LORD while in a foreign land?' I believe the answer is 'Because we must not forget.' In the despair of depression, in an exile brought about by a mental health crisis, we forget the place from where we have travelled. That there was once a time of laughter, love, enjoyment and happiness becomes a memory that is difficult and painful to grasp. The need is for companions who will bear our pain, endure our anger and, as they sit alongside us by that unfamiliar river, sing songs of remembrance, songs of hope and songs that remind us of the people we are. I value my friends who can sit alongside me in the place of lament. They are few, but they are trusted companions who do not offer me their wisdom, advice, encouragement, instruction, but instead sit with me beside the river and offer me a silent companionship of presence, and in that they speak powerfully of the presence and consistency of God's love. That I am not abandoned in my despair is a powerful counter to the inner voice that says I am nothing, I am worthless.

Recovering the power of lament is an urgent task for communities of faith. It takes great patience to sit, in love, alongside someone who is unable to love themselves. It takes great courage to be with the one who is a stranger to you, whose behaviour and words stir fear and uncertainty within you. It requires a continual commitment in prayer and reliance upon the Spirit, seeking to look upon the heart and not the outward appearance; to look beyond the immediate and see the journey travelled and the road ahead. It also requires those of you who are companions to people living in despair to look after yourself. 'Love your neighbour as yourself,' Jesus said. Self-care isn't self-indulgence, placing yourself and your inner life before that of others. Self-care is knowing that in order to love those who cannot love themselves, you need to be continuously restored through the love of Christ, knowing rest and peace where the demand of the despair of others isn't present.

I used to hate my wife going away. I'd mope about the place, feel miserable, throw myself into whatever work I had with ever greater commitment, drink as soon as I arrived home to numb the feeling of the emptiness of an empty home. It took me a long time to realize that the ability of despair and depression to turn me in on myself made me an utterly selfish person. I was miserable because I was alone, because my wife hadn't put me first, that her absence from me was because I wasn't worthy of her presence. It was all about me, which is ironic, as I didn't like me!

Marriage is a gift. I never anticipated that I would marry, but when I met my wife we were both single students in the first year of theological college, training for ministry. From the moment I saw her I loved her. I'd never thought I would be capable of such a depth of certainty and emotion. My wife had been praying to meet a man who was honest, and on our first date I was honest about my life and its challenges. I thought it better to be honest from the start and to give this amazing woman the chance to run for the hills! But she listened to a young man's honesty, we were engaged eight weeks later, and married ten months after our first meeting. Marriage is a gift, and during our marriage I have discovered it is all too easy to take a gift for granted; to take a person's presence and love for granted, to expect them to evidence endless reserves of love and compassion, to be always understanding, always patient, always gentle, always attentive to me and my needs.

I have been a very selfish man in my despair. 'My God, my God, why have you forsaken me?' The opening words of the psalmist in Psalm 22 were to echo down the centuries, to be spoken again by the Word made flesh as he hung nailed to a Roman cross, a cry of utter anguish spoken out by the Word into creation. The psalmist continues: 'Why are you so far from saving me, so far from my cries of anguish?' In my marriage I thought any distance from my wife was a sign of abandonment, but this was the projection of a young boy fearful and humiliated, despairing at the loneliness and isolation that had once again enfolded him. My wife is not my saviour, but she is a gift from my Saviour, a companion in life as we journey home heavenward together.

Her reserves of love are not endless, her compassion is not without limits, and she is in as much need of patience, kindness and gentleness as any other person. I used to place her upon a saintly pedestal of being my saviour in life and then feel angry and frustrated when she couldn't meet my needs.

My wife is the Saviour's gift to me, a loving companion who sits by the fire with me when all others have gone home, tired of the conversation, exhausted by my exhaustion. Full of a wisdom, compassion and hope that has come from years spent in mission, seeing people come to Christ, seeing people come off heroin in Hong Kong, seeing lives in different parts of the world transformed by Jesus. My wife knows that Jesus is her Saviour, and in order to be able to love me and offer me compassion she needs time when it is about her care and recovery and not mine. And so I've had to learn to temper despair, to put fear aside, to quieten anger and enable my wife to have her time of care, her time of peace, to be listened to and offered compassion, and understand that this is my gift and my duty to her. For my wife, self-care is dinner out with an old friend, time away with trusted friends, time to laugh and time to simply be in Christ's presence; time without despair.

Chapter note

In this chapter I've written of the experience of suicide and suicidal ideation. If you have experienced, or are currently experiencing, thoughts of ending your life through suicide, or are imagining your death and how to die, please contact the Samaritans at www.samaritans.org. *If you are in the UK, you can also call them on 116 123.*

5

Surrender

A year after becoming a Christian I was attending a local church and had been invited on a church weekend away. It was a wonderful time of laughter, prayer, friendship and family. Experience of the different church families I encountered was teaching me how to relate and how to trust. Of course, being a church weekend away, there was the usual schedule of worship, teaching, prayer and ministry.

Everything had been going fine until the final morning session before we all returned home. As part of the session there was a time of prayer, and a friend's mother came up to me and asked if she could pray for me. I agreed. She placed her hand on my shoulder, began to pray and then suddenly stopped. There was a moment of silence, then she began to pray for me again, only to stop once more a few moments later. As a new Christian I wasn't sure if this was normal and quite what I was meant to do. I was also wondering what on earth this woman was going to pray for, if she kept stopping every time she tried to pray for me. Was God revealing some hideous sin in me? Was she so utterly shocked that she had no idea what to pray, or how to exit the space without anyone noticing? My good old paranoia had kicked in on full power, and in the silence I was now wondering how on earth I could move away from this woman, who still had her hand on my shoulder, and pretend to anyone looking that I had no idea what this nutcase was doing; she clearly needed retraining in how to pray for people.

It was at the moment of preparing to break away that she spoke to me.

'I'm sorry, Rob, but it's very strange. Every time I pray for you . . .'

Silence again.

'Yes,' I replied desperately, trying to avoid my 'yes' sounding like a question inviting more detail.

'I'm sorry, but every time I pray for you . . .'

Yet more silence . . . hand still on shoulder.

'Yes!' Perhaps an affirmation of her desire to pray for me would somehow end this.

'Every time I pray for you, it is strange, you see, but every time I pray for you I see an old man.'

Okay, an 'old man'; that was a first, that had my interest, 'Yes?'

'Every time I pray for you I see an old man who is bent over from the weight of all he is carrying.'

'Ah.' The image wasn't a surprise.

'The old man is bent over because he is carrying great rocks and they weigh him down.'

'Hmmm . . .' I was playing for time and an opportunity to end the conversation.

'It is strange, because when I close my eyes I see an old man, but when I open my eyes I see a young man. It simply doesn't make any sense to me. You're a young man! You're 18! How can you be old and burdened! I'm sorry, my prayer isn't helpful.'

And there was the opening to end this. 'It is very strange. Doesn't sound like me at all. Thank you so much for being willing to pray for me. I guess sometimes our prayer wires get a bit crossed!'

I took my opportunity, left the room and found a quiet space outside away from everyone. I was angry, fearful, ashamed and despairing that God not only knew my innermost being but that he would make what was hidden known to someone else. This action on God's part was outrageous to me. How could he betray what was hidden?

Where can I go from your Spirit?
Where can I flee from your presence?

I'm not sure David intended me to declare his words in Psalm 139 as a statement of frustration rather than a declaration of hope, but why is God so 'God'? I mean, why can't God be a bit less 'God in your face'. Why must he be so darn relentlessly compassionate? You see, when you've survived abuse or trauma, the compassion of another can be painful; an expression of love can be physically impossible to receive because it might not be compassion or love, it might simply be a means to an end. Worse than that, to be offered compassion or love is to be offered that which tears open an old festering wound and allows someone to poke about in deeply painful places. For children who are trauma survivors, it is not unusual for a 'Well done for . . .' or 'I'm really proud of you for . . .' to lead to an act of violence as the child rejects the pain of feeling loved or cared for. I know this feeling as an adult, when you want to put out of sight that for which you have received love or compassion because it is never enough to fill the void of love and compassion that exists deep within.

For years I've received thank-you cards from people, either after speaking at an event, taking a funeral or a wedding, from students who I've taught and nurtured through training for ministry. Each card is a beautiful expression of another person's affection, love and appreciation. But for many years each card has been both painful and beautiful in equal measure. Early in ministry I couldn't read the cards, but at the same time I couldn't throw them away because I valued the fact that this was another person's gift to me, and that gift held the value of their time and thankfulness. I would simply put them away in a box, stored safely behind a set of drawers where no one could find them and where I could never see them.

> For you created my inmost being;
>> you knit me together in my mother's womb.
> I praise you because I am fearfully and
>> wonderfully made;
>> your works are wonderful,
>> I know that full well.
> (Psalm 139.13–14)

Studying theology has been a saving act for me. It has saved me from the reliance on my otherwise unreliable emotions. My innermost being may feel utterly shame-filled, I may resent my very existence, I may despair at how I have been made and broken, I may reject the beauty of all that surrounds me, but I know full well that nothing I can say, do, scream, reject or deny can change the unalterable action of God's extravagantly loving activity in creation. God can't be any less God, regardless of my frustration, because God is God and that God is God is utterly sufficient.

But here is the heart of the matter: God surrendered all. The Word became flesh and made his dwelling among us. The Word that spoke all that is seen and unseen into being, humbled himself, became a man and lived among us. He was not less than God, for he was God,

who, being in very nature God,
    did not consider equality with God
        something to be used to his own advantage;
rather, he made himself nothing
    by taking the very nature of a servant,
    being made in human likeness.
And being found in appearance as a man,
    he humbled himself by becoming obedient to
        death –
    even death on a cross!
(Philippians 2.6–8)

These words from Paul in Philippians are with me every day. Every day I marvel at Christ's obedience, his love, his willingness to surrender all to save all.

Obedience has been the one consistent aspect of my faith in Jesus from the very first moment I met him. He said 'Follow', and I followed; simple really. However, surrender has taken a rather longer time to develop in my life. You see,

I liked my rocks. I knew what life was like, feeling old before my time, feeling burdened by memory and pain. The weight of pain in my life was a familiar old friend. I knew fear, shame, anger, despair. I knew them well, and the thought of putting them down, of leaving them behind, was painful, almost too awful to imagine. Surrendering to what is familiar is a darn sight easier than surrendering to what is unfamiliar, and as an 18-year-old, I had no intention of surrendering what I knew.

What I hadn't realized at that point in my life was that I had already surrendered. I had surrendered hope, love, joy; I had surrendered my horizon because I was bent double looking at the floor carrying my familiar friends. Furthermore, and perhaps what has shocked me most as I have grown older, there was the realization that I had surrendered to pride and not to humility. I thought that carrying my own burden and not placing it on others was the greatest expression of Christian humility – turns out it was just plain ignorant pride. I was proud of my ability to carry my rocks. I'd done it, no one else, no one had helped me, this was all my own work of bloody-minded survival, and the fear-fuelled, shame-surviving, anger-agitated, despair-driven, sheer hard work of simply living had kept me alive! Only it hadn't. It hadn't kept me alive; it had kept me existing and in doing so had consumed my childhood and was slowly consuming my adulthood until there would be nothing left and no reason to continue.

The journey of surrender would begin a year later. I'd left school aged 18 having successfully failed to achieve my A-level grades (and in one case any A-level at all) and in

God's good grace found myself working for an organization called Mencap Homes Foundation, supporting people with learning disabilities to live within a community-based home. It was a time of hard lessons and great satisfaction; it was also a time when my inability to react well when triggered by a person or event found full exposure. My PTSD had been triggered by the actions of another, and my Shield Against Shame response had been anger, which I'd written down in a staff handover book. The book was meant to enable one staff shift to note down key events and needs for the next staff shift; it was an important communication tool. However, I'd decided to use it to express the full flight of my anger about the attitude of others. This in turn triggered responses by other members of staff, angered by my public airing of my anger, and escalated the whole situation.

At the next staff meeting the use of the handover book was discussed, and in the meeting a deputy manager was very clear about what she thought about my attitude and behaviour towards others. As I heard her words my shame took flight as my humiliation deepened. Feelings of fear, anger and despair started to overwhelm me, the room began to close in, it grew difficult to breathe, I felt light-headed, I felt as though I was being trapped, that the people sitting around me were about to harm me. There was no escape: I had to run. The deputy manager finished speaking, I made my excuses and left the room. I went to the toilet furthest away from the staff meeting, locked the door and cried. Ashamed, terrified, a small boy who had no idea what to do next.

Over the next few weeks my emotions became increasingly unreliable, tears welled up at the thought of going into work, I had difficulty sleeping, I felt permanently exhausted, my concentration was shot and my paranoia was firing on all cylinders. I don't know what made me go to my doctor, but I did. I remember sitting in the consulting room with him, he explained what a breakdown was, asked me about my mental health, and offered me a choice: tablets or talking therapy. I chose talking therapy, and a month or so later I was sitting in a room with a man who was explaining what a therapist was and asked me about my life, the incident at work and what it reminded me of. Without realizing, I'd entered the place of surrender.

Our call is not simply to surrender the rocks of trauma that we carry in our lives, it is to surrender our lives to and in Christ; it is the surrender of our story, in all its gruesome detail. For as we surrender our story to Jesus, we are caught up in his story, a story of rescue, redemption, of hope renewed. What I was to discover was that Jesus is not ashamed of my story, for in him it is made new. At the end of six months of talking therapy I'd finally told someone one part of my story. I was beginning to understand how the story of my past had written the story of my present and was trying to write the story of my future. I'd only told part of my story, but not because I intentionally held the full story back. More accurately, now I see that God in his grace has been renewing my story in Christ, one chapter at a time, and in that grace I have not been overwhelmed even when the greatest storms of trauma have raged within me.

As I write this, I'm reminded of a gift of God's compassion I had forgotten. At the end of the six months of talking therapy, which had taken place at my local adult mental health centre, in the final session the therapist, who had patiently listened, reflected and enabled me to connect, explained that he had particularly asked for my case file from all the various ones available. He was a Christian and had felt called to be my therapist. Gifts of heaven are very, very precious.

However, surrender is a lifelong journey, for our stories are made up of our long-lived lives. I've reconciled myself to the fact that it can feel as though I revisit the same story in different contexts. Lived trauma is wired into our brains and constantly affects how we narrate and experience life. Time and again my past crashes into my present, attempting to erase what God has been writing in my life.

Entering rural ministry in my late thirties was to once again trigger past memory. In 2010, I had started a new post as rector of seven rural parishes. They were located in stunning countryside and I loved pottering between the people and parishes, driving along quiet country roads, encountering visitors in the different churches, enjoying the views from hilltops. It was the first time I'd lived in the countryside in nearly 20 years and memories were stirring inside me, my anxiety was gradually building, and for some reason I'd started to fear where I'd been called to serve.

The Book of Common Prayer service of Holy Communion is a rich and beautiful service. It has a careful rhythm of language that carries you. I was presiding at one of the seven parish churches, which had a wonderful history. People had worshipped on the site for over a thousand years, and on a summer's morning we would open up a side door allowing sunlight and birdsong, and the sound of the odd sheep or two, to stream into the chancel where we would gather for our early morning communion.

It was then that my past decided to gatecrash my present once again. In the midst of the service, as I was speaking the words of the service over bread and wine, I glimpsed the light pouring through the door, the shadow of a tree on the tiled floor, the birdsong flooding in, and at that moment I wasn't standing at a communion table, I was being abused; there in the beauty of creation I was once again feeling my body touched, the ground pressing beneath me. I felt utterly alone and afraid.

I should have expected it: a few days earlier I'd had a similar experience. Walking to a meeting in the evening dusk I'd passed by one of the primary schools I served, and, as I walked past, dusk turned to day and I was standing at the gate of my old primary school, a familiar fear rising within me. That evening I'd closed my eyes, shaken my head, reminded myself where I was, and walked on to my meeting. At the communion service the physical sensation of abuse caught me utterly unawares. I completed the service, and left.

Learning to surrender has taken me a long time. You'd have thought that after years of therapy, medication and prayer I'd have known by now what to do, but instead I did what was familiar. Fear gripped me; in my anger I pushed those closest away. I wanted to hide my shame, and despair, good old despair, gradually sucked all hope from my mind, leaving suicide as once again the best option available. In the midst of the approaching breakdown, my wife, once again recognizing the signs, stepped in to secure the treatment I needed; treatment that was finally to give me the tools to understand my story fully and to surrender with confidence to the one who loved me.

Now almost ten years later, surrender is my life's goal. My desire is that there should be ever less of me and ever more of Christ within. I'm slowly discovering the journey of kenosis, of self-emptying that Paul describes in the second chapter of Philippians I am gradually realizing that when Paul wrote, 'What is more, I consider everything a loss because of the surpassing worth of knowing Christ Jesus my Lord, for whose sake I have lost all things' (Philippians 3.8), that the surrender of my story is a joyous surrender to the one who surrendered heaven for the sake of love. Our journey of surrender is not a downward spiral of being emptied but an upward dance to take hold of the one who has taken hold of us, Christ Jesus.

6

Forgiveness

In 2018 we were sitting in a classroom at the Kigali Genocide Memorial Museum. It was the start of our journey in Rwanda and we had yet to meet the man who would talk of his father's murderer, and forgiveness, and the murderer of his father who would talk of the work of reconciliation. Having spent time in the memorial, Revd Dr Antoine Rutayisire, a survivor of the genocide who served as a Commissioner on the National Unity and Reconciliation Commission, explained his story of survival, of reconciliation, of hope, and explained that, in the aftermath of the Rwandan genocide in which nearly one million people were killed in approximately three months, the realization had come to him that the forgiveness that would be needed was to be found in the words of Jesus on the cross, from Luke's Gospel: 'Father, forgive them, for they do not know what they are doing' (Luke 23.34).

I found this breathtaking. I had spent the afternoon in the Kigali Genocide Memorial learning about the abhorrent violence one person can commit against another. I'd seen the skulls of those killed, the machete marks clearly visible. This was brutal, ugly violence in its most disgusting perverted form, and yet a man who is respected nationally and internationally, who survived this bloody murder, whose family was directly affected by it, was able to look to Christ and see the beginning of forgiveness. I was left reeling at the shallowness of my understanding. I was completely thrown that this man, that a nation, had found in Jesus a remarkable reconciliation that had been slowly but surely rebuilding hope in the midst of the blood of a million men, women and children.

It turns out forgiveness is not my thing. I always thought it was. I thought I had forgiveness nailed, until that day at the Genocide Memorial and the compassion-filled words of a man who survived. I thought I was a 'forgive and forget' kind of person, that all the therapy and prayer had enabled me really to get to grips with forgiveness. Quick to forgive, quick to keep no record of wrongs, quick to simply get on with life. To some extent that is true. I am able to forgive people, and I know that because I know I have forgiven people, but if I'm honest, this has been forgiveness on a small scale, forgiveness for thoughtlessness, forgiveness for actions or inaction, forgiveness for words spoken or not spoken. This kind of forgiveness makes it easy to 'forget', to move on and to keep moving.

But the forgiveness that Antoine was describing was forgiveness born out of profound lasting trauma.

'Father, forgive them, for they do not know what they are doing.' I had noticed this before, but I'd been skipping the second part of Jesus' statement, 'for they do not know what they are doing'. I'd been able to reflect upon it theologically; I understood that this was the Son speaking to the Father of the ignorance of humanity, unaware that they were murdering the one who had spoken them into being, unaware that in this act of murder the redemption and reconciliation of creation to its Creator would be enacted. I'd also reflected on the context of these words, only to be found in Luke's Gospel and not in some earlier manuscripts of it, as the phrase could have been added by later Roman converts. But I'd never taken those words and placed them into the lived world. I'd never allowed them beyond the interaction of the Godhead, between Son and Father, allowed them to affect how I understand and live out forgiveness in all its fullness. Those who nailed Christ to the cross were like me, blinded by sin and shame to the reality of the Father's love.

It turns out forgiveness is not my thing. What I long to do is forget. I want to forgive in order to be able to forget, to leave behind the past because surely leaving behind the past is what it means to experience a form of spiritual freedom? However, this freedom is false, it is insecure, it lasts until the next trigger of trauma or memory, the next time the Shield Against Shame is put into action, and there it is, the same old hurt, the same familiar pain. In that familiarity confusion creeps in as you look at the pain and at the situation, and in frustration cry, 'But I've dealt with this. I've forgiven. Why do I need to forgive again and again and again?' My lesson in Rwanda was that forgiveness without the reconciliation that comes through the understanding of 'other' is merely a sticking plaster, a shallow imitation of a forgiveness that is life-transforming.

It is too easy in our contemporary world to translate forgiveness as primarily an individualized feeling; forgiving another as some form of 'thought exercise', which is ultimately one-sided. It is my forgiveness of you, which is not dependent upon action on your part or any requirement for me to understand what I am forgiving you for. However, in Jesus' context, forgiveness was enacted, intentional, it involved a physical act. Forgiveness was enacted reciprocity, 'as you have been forgiven', a point that Paul makes in his letters to the churches in Ephesus and Colossae. This was the kind of forgiveness that was lived out, enabling communities to resolve conflict, find ways to live in Christ with one another, and continue to offer the extravagant love of God made known in Christ. This is what it means to be part of the body of Christ, a body made up of vastly different people bound together by a common Saviour; forgiveness is an act of community, not merely that of an individual.

As a survivor of abuse, I find this call to forgiveness, forgiveness that is enacted, not simply spoken but lived out, to be profoundly challenging. In Christ I am forgiven; totally, completely, utterly forgiven. Yet as a someone who is still bound to this mortal and frail life I am still subject to my history, to the effect of sin, to the stickiness of shame. As Christians we continuously live lives of profound tension, the tension between the kingdom that has come and is coming and the kingdom that is passing away; the tension between life and death, between mortality and eternity, between what was and is and what will be. We cannot escape this, and it is a tension that shapes our experience of forgiveness and our ability to forgive. '"Holy, holy, holy is the Lord God Almighty," who was, and is, and is to come' is the cry from Revelation 4. 'Who was, and is, and is to come' is a beautiful description of the landscape of our lives as Christians, a landscape that holds the tension of past, present and future, and therefore one in which I shouldn't be surprised when forgiveness is an act that requires all three aspects of that landscape to be enacted in order to bring completion.

What struck me time and again in Rwanda was the way survivors would speak of how perpetrators had been shaped by the violent intention of others, and the way perpetrators would describe their horror at the violence they had committed, the way they hadn't understood what they were doing, their fear of the retaliation of survivors and their surprise at the grace in which communities had received them back. This picture of forgiveness and reconciliation isn't complete or perfect in Rwanda: there are still many who harbour violence, many who are unable to forgive. But in those I met, those who had walked this hard journey of reconciling past, present and future enacted in forgiveness, in those people I saw freedom: a freedom to hope, to love, to live with one another, and to build lives together; that is the evidence of the power of forgiveness – communities transformed.

However, this forgiveness didn't mean forgetting. It didn't mean airbrushing history to make out that because we're all friends now nothing really happened. Perhaps that is the importance of the Genocide Memorials in Rwanda. It is the importance of visiting, or listening, of learning from the lived experience of others; it means we cannot forget.

Nyamata Genocide Memorial Centre has at its heart a church. In 1994, as the genocide began, ten thousand people shut themselves in the church in the hope of finding sanctuary. All ten thousand were slaughtered in the church, the evidence of their deaths still plain to see today. About fifty thousand were killed in the Nyamata area, and many of their remains are held in coffins contained in a series of catacomb-like structures underground next to the church. On the day of our visit to Nyamata, all of us were uncertain about entering the underground chambers, knowing that we were on sacred ground that had been soaked by the blood of thousands of people. I found myself moving forward and stepping on to the walkway that led underground; it is perhaps the closest I will ever come to 'descending into death'. The mausoleum was a simple, white-tiled, clean, respectful place with coffin upon coffin stacked with the skeletal remains of men, women and children. Some had photographs put close to them, in the hope that somewhere in this chamber their loved one's remains were safe. At the end of our visit a young man, who had accompanied us around the Memorial and had offered time and explanations to us, thanked us for giving our time to visit and to listen. As the rest of our party got ready to go, I wanted to thank him for his time and care for us and found him in his office gently leaning against a wall, his head bowed, breathing carefully. He was a child at the time of Nyamata, his home was in Nyamata, and he had somehow survived the slaughter of the genocide. He explained that enabling visitors to remember the story of Nyamata and the power of forgiveness and reconciliation was important, because in not forgetting there was much to be learnt and much to be thankful for. But each time he retold the story of Nyamata he retold the story of his own profound and violent trauma. It was a privilege to meet a young man who had such a sense of call to hold in tension his past and present, at great personal cost, in order to ensure that lessons were remembered that could shape a better future for others.

It turns out forgiveness is a lifelong act. I came back from Rwanda changed. I realized the shallowness of the forgiveness I had enacted; I realized the challenge of the forgiveness Christ calls us to live out. 'Father, forgive them, for they do not know what they are doing.'

Did the two people who abused me know what they were doing? Did those who bullied me to the point of my wanting to end my life know what they were doing? Perhaps the lesson I am discovering from Rwanda is that the answer is yes and no and maybe. Yes, they harmed me directly, caught up in the immediacy of their actions. No, they couldn't have foreseen the outcome of their actions upon me. Maybe they should have or could have, but I don't know and I can't live second-guessing the 'why' of what someone did. I know that the teacher who harmed me changed after getting married, and became gentle, even kind – which was very strange at the time. I know that the other person who abused me was in a family facing profound trauma and had many fears. I know that the children who bullied me had complex family lives, which I learnt more of as I discovered more about the community in which we lived.

These things I know, and in that 'knowing' I'm discovering there is a Jesus-made space to begin to understand, to begin to be reconciled, to begin to imagine meeting the person and offering that person the grace I have been given in Jesus.

I realize that for some people I am undermining justice. I risk taking on the responsibility and shame of others, which is not mine to take. I know that for some the thought of forgiveness being rooted in the understanding of others will be an anathema to be resisted, because it risks undermining their journey of healing. I know this because people have said all of this to me.

And yet, and yet, in Christ I am forgiven. I am forgiven and Jesus knows me fully, every little bit of me. My identity is not simply that of a 'survivor': I have sinned and fallen short of the glory of God like everybody else. I've hurt people, I've caused harm, I've intentionally acted against others, I've responded in anger, with hatred, I've closed people out of my life and rejected people. But I know that before Christ Jesus, my Saviour and Redeemer, I cannot point the finger to my past and say 'It's all their fault' and in doing so pin the blame of my sin and shame upon others as I cry, 'They made me who I am.'

No. God made me who I am, a man made to be in relationship with him, but a man separated from that relationship by the effect of sin and shame; the sin and shame of others, the corruption of creation, and the sin and shame that is my own and no one else's. And in truth, the hardest person I find to forgive is myself. For from the scars of my trauma, my innermost being cries out at all the ways I have failed, all the ways I am hateful, all the ways I am unforgiveable; a man of shame, formed by shame, in whom shame is found. Forgiveness is hard when you do not know how to forgive yourself.

Praise the LORD, my soul;
    all my inmost being, praise his holy name.
Praise the LORD, my soul,
    and forget not all his benefits –
who forgives all your sins
    and heals all your diseases,

who redeems your life from the pit
    and crowns you with love and compassion,
who satisfies your desires with good things
    so that your youth is renewed like the eagle's.
(Psalm 103.1–5)

The adventure of faith has brought many benefits. The fact that I am alive, that an angry, fear-ridden, shame-filled young man didn't take his own life is a remarkable gift for which I will be for ever grateful. The renewal of my life has meant I have lived to be able to love, hope, trust and learn how to forgive. I am living a life that has been renewed like the eagle's. I cannot forget what God has done in Christ Jesus. I cannot deny his presence or his love, just as I cannot deny what has taken place in my life. What I can do is this: living in the forgiveness of Christ, I can seek the reconciliation of past, present and future, that I may know what it is to live reconciled to all that was, is and will be.

Jesus is the ultimate act of enacted forgiveness. The Father didn't simply pronounce forgiveness over all creation, he enacted forgiveness in himself through the Son, the creative Word of God, who spoke all things seen and unseen into being, who was obedient to death, even death on a cross,

as far as the east is from the west,
    so far has he removed our transgressions from us.
(Psalm 103.12)

This pilgrim remains a work in progress. To surrender to forgiveness feels like an odd call, but it is real and evident in my life. There is much that I have yet to surrender and much that I do not understand or know. I still carry trauma. I still remember. I still don't know how I would act if I were to meet my perpetrators. I still experience depression and anxiety. Post-traumatic stress disorder is still a part of my life. I still remain thankful for the skills of therapists and scientists who form medications that bring relief when despair has taken hold. I am still learning how to forgive myself.

I am grateful to the people I met in Rwanda, for the generosity of their time, their words, their actions. I travelled there as a man who didn't realize the poverty of his understanding. I returned enriched in discovering that if we can live in forgiveness, true Jesus-enabled forgiveness, not the forgive-and-forget kind, but the forgive-and-be-reconciled kind, then the fruit of that reconciliation flows ever richer as it is caught up in the reconciliation of Creator and creation in Christ Jesus, renewing our lives, our communities and our world.

7

Faith

Having written about the need to persevere in faith, the writer of the letter to the Hebrews reflected: 'Now faith is confidence in what we hope for and assurance about what we do not see. This is what the ancients were commended for' (Hebrews 11.1–2). The writer then goes on to recount stories of faith that were ground into the lived experience of the Jewish people.

Stories of faith are a vital resource in sustaining confidence and assurance as we make our journey through life. Stories of others are helpful, but just as important are our own stories of faith. Our stories of how we encountered Jesus and followed him are the bedrock of our faithfulness in living out our calling. I wonder how many times the first followers in the earliest days of the Church recounted their stories of Jesus? Stories to encourage one another, to nurture and uphold. Stories to remind them who they were in the midst of great challenge and persecution. Those stories were gifts to be shared among the community of believers.

One of the things I encourage people to do is to share their stories of Jesus; to tell each other their story of faith, because in retelling their story they recall again the love of Jesus and encourage their own continued faithfulness. You can tell when the disease of individualization has infected a church community: nobody knows each other's story of faith. The wonder of our stories is that each one is different; there are often familiar themes in our common humanity, but Jesus calls each of us as we are. My wife's story is one of growing up in a Christian family, of knowing the constancy of Jesus in her life, of seeing Jesus transform the lives of others through prayer and knowing him deeply and richly. My story is one of a young man who needed an enormous spiritual kick up the backside, which he received, if he was ever going to notice anything but his own anger and pain. These stories hold who we are in Jesus, they are the stories of our birth in Jesus, and they are there to be shared.

Living as I do with a long-term mental health condition, my story of faith has been a constant foundation stone that I return to again and again. When God seems far and faith appears absent, I return to the story of when Jesus first called me to follow him, and something in me starts to beat my heart to heaven's rhythm once again. When I'm numb in the midst of depression, when despair has vacuumed all hope from me and there seems to be nothing left, there is still the reality of my story. In years gone by, when thoughts of suicide have filled my mind, I haven't been able to shake my story, which tells me that in death my Saviour will wonder what I'm doing before him when he hadn't called me yet.

I write 'my story', but the story isn't mine. In fact, none of our stories are our own. All of our stories are part of the story of God; my story caught up in the wonder that is his story, a story of his grace, mercy and how he makes himself known to us in the fullness and extravagance of his love when we least expect it. That's the story that is revealed throughout Scripture. It is the story made known in the Incarnation. It is the story the Church proclaims; the Creator who is love so loves his creation that he has stepped in to rescue and return to relationship the whole of creation. All of this is God's activity, not ours. We have to crawl on and carry off parts in the most extravagant story of love in all eternity, the story of God.

When I was younger, I thought God was a fairy tale, a fiction made up for weak people to keep them weak. I was 16, I'd survived this far in life, and no god or God was going to be able to claim any credit for my hard work. I'd survived by shutting down and keeping myself numb to feelings of love or compassion. What I did feel was fear, shame, anger and despair. Although you wouldn't have spotted them, I'd figured out a long time ago that they were the power station in my life; they fuelled my resilience and bloody-minded determination; they were mine and no one was going to take them from me. I'd told my story once when I was 12 to a therapist. I received a summer of intensive speech therapy and as part of that I'd been filmed and asked by two therapists why I thought I had a speech impediment. I'd told them about one of my abusers, I'd told them about the trauma of seeing my sister attacked by a dog, I'd told them about the bullying and how it made me feel that I wanted to die. They'd filmed me and nothing changed. No adult took any notice, nothing was said to my parents; my life had simply passed by unnoticed, and that was how I'd decided it was going to stay.

I still have no idea why on earth I thought it was a good idea to attend the sixth form of the town's local grammar school. I was the only boy from my secondary school to apply in my year. The friends I'd made at secondary school were applying to go to local colleges and, with my ability to shut down emotions, any feelings of loss about my friends were non-existent. Reflecting as an adult, I might have wanted the status of attending the local grammar school. What I actually got was a whole lot more bullying; it turned out the boys at the grammar school didn't like the idea of a boy from the secondary school attending. It was only after I started that I discovered the last boy to attempt it had been bullied out of the school after a term. Still, not being liked was familiar territory, being shunned felt normal, and the physical threats were no worse than anything I'd survived before; my power station was running well.

What was different this time was a bunch of Christian boys in the sixth form. They were particularly annoying. I knew what it was like not to be liked. However, the Christians were nice, they were interested, they were likeable, and they kept on talking about Jesus.

Talking about Jesus was particularly infuriating. I was infuriated because they were lying. They were talking about a mythical figure as if he was real, delusional souls that they were. Worse than that, they were encouraging people to believe in this mythical figure as if he was some kind of answer to the questions of humanity. Lies, upon lies, upon lies. I put up with it in my first term at the school because I was too busy surviving the onslaught of bullying. But in the second term, I'd had enough and went to the headmaster of the school to complain. The headmaster listened to my complaint about these Christians who told lies and were delusional, and politely dismissed my concerns, much to my consternation.

The Christians continued to talk about Jesus and continued to be 'nice'. I continued to endure them and publicly tell them what delusional idiots they were whenever I could. Until one day when they actually invited me to a Christian Union meeting. Full credit to them for perseverance; I was not an easy invite!

However, my survival instinct has always been based on a deep pragmatism. The day they invited me happened to be on a particularly cold and wet day. As a boy's school you all had to go outside during break times. I think it was meant to be good for us, though I've no idea what frostbite or pneumonia adds to life. I knew that the Christian Union meeting was held in the nice, warm, dry woodwork room. I also knew that hot chocolate was served at the end of a Christian Union meeting. My pragmatism kicked in and the Christian boys were delighted when I said I would attend their meeting.

I can still remember sitting there, listening to the talk about Jesus, and thinking to myself what utter rubbish I was hearing. I can remember thinking how weak they were as I happily consumed my hot chocolate, so weak that they had to believe in some kind of higher power to enable them to get through a day. On the way back across the school grounds after the meeting, one of the boys excitedly asked what I thought about what I had heard. My response was very clear: 'You are all nutters. Someone should lock you up and throw away the key. Never invite me to one of your meetings again.' As I mentioned earlier, I was a challenging invite.

The Christians left me alone for the rest of the term. Life was peaceful, the bullying had subsided with the help of a kind teacher, who was highly regarded in the school and who had taken me under his wing. He took time each week to walk with me in the school grounds and listen to my experiences in the school. What I discovered later was that he also took each of my tormentors to one side and told them they would not be welcomed in the school any longer if they continued in their actions. Easter arrived, the Spring term began, and brought with it a period of cold and wet weather – and my pragmatism. Standing outside in the cold and rain is not much fun when you know there is a room that is warm, dry and in which hot chocolate is available. The only downside was the Christians in the room. However, on one particular day the Christian boys in the sixth form were not about, so I seized the opportunity for warmth and hot chocolate.

When I entered the woodwork room I made sure I sat in a corner away from the Christian nutcases. My only interest was being warm and the hot chocolate that was to come. The Christians had their Christian Union meeting, someone talked about Jesus (again), but the unusual thing this time was that someone offered to lead a prayer of commitment. Apparently, if anyone wanted to 'give their life to Jesus' they could pray this prayer of commitment, become a Christian and Jesus would be with them. This caught my interest. I suddenly realized I had a unique opportunity to prove them all wrong, to catch them out in their lies. I knew God was a fake. So I determined to say their 'prayer of commitment', but that at the end of it I would lift up my head and laugh at them, because there was no God, there was no mythical Jesus, and they were all fools. I didn't tell anyone what I was doing; it was my little experiment that couldn't go wrong.

However, I thought to myself that if I was going to say the prayer and carry out my experiment, I would say the prayer properly. That turned out to be my last thought as a non-Christian.

As I said the prayer, three things happened to me. First of all, I had what I can only describe as a vision. I didn't know it was a 'vision' at the time, I just thought it was weird. I had a vision that I was standing on the edge of an abyss. The abyss was deep and dark, and I stepped off the edge into it. As I stepped off and started to fall, two hands came up out of the abyss and caught me.

If that wasn't strange enough, the second thing happened. As the hands caught me, I had a strange warm, fuzzy sensation from my head to my toes, like being in a warm bath, utterly immersive and utterly peaceful.

And then the third and really strange thing happened. The vision and warm fuzzy feeling had come as a bit of a surprise, so I opened my eyes. Except when I opened my eyes I didn't see the woodwork room, I saw an incredibly bright blinding light that forced me to close my eyes. I opened my eyes again and sat there blinking, surprised, shocked, looking around for the rotter who had just shone a torch in my eyes, but there was no one near me, I was on my own in the corner of the room. I looked for the sun glaring off a car windscreen in the teachers' car park opposite, but it was a wet and cloudy day; there was no sunshine. I can still remember blinking and leaving the woodwork room. I didn't tell anyone in the room what had just happened.

I didn't *know* what had just happened. Then the thought struck me as I was walking back to class for the start of that afternoon's lessons. I had been accusing the Christians of being liars, but if I denied what had just happened to me, I would become the liar.

The rest of the afternoon was spent blinking and thinking. Whatever the bright light had been it had affected my eyesight, and even dark corners in dimly lit rooms seemed to shimmer with a light. I spent my afternoon in a history lesson, sitting in a small dimly lit library room, not daring to tell any of my five other classmates what had just happened to me.

Later that day my mum asked me how my day had been. My response was a bewildered, 'I think I might have become a Christian.'

Now, I'm writing a book about trauma and mental health and as part of the book I am telling my story. Don't think you're the first one to wonder if my experience that day in the woodwork room was some kind of psychosis; I wondered it long before you. I've wondered if I had some kind of psychotic episode, some form of manic experience that meant I became in some way disembodied and observed myself externally. As a lecturer and researcher in mental health and spirituality later in my life, I can assure you I have called into question with great detail every aspect of that afternoon. But I was calm and I wasn't distressed. I wasn't hospitalized or manic from the episode. I wasn't distressed or anxious prior to the experience or after the experience. I'd attended Sunday school as a child, and while I'd played with fuzzy-felt and drawn pictures, I have no recollection of any story that could have informed or shaped my experience subconsciously. I couldn't explain it. Well, I could explain it, but the explanation was inconvenient and profoundly challenging: God had shown me he was real and I was the deluded one thinking that he wasn't.

Having encouraged the sharing of our stories of faith, I must now admit that I've rarely shared my story. It isn't that I'm embarrassed or unsure of it. It is simply that I know that it has a drama to it and I know it wasn't the solution to all my problems. It isn't that I look back and hope that it had been some kind of spiritual lobotomy that flicked a switch in my brain for ever, removing my memories of trauma – though that would have been nice. It is that my story has been of fundamental meaning to me. It was the start of a remarkable journey in which an extraordinary love entered my life in the person of Jesus, and perhaps my fear in sharing my story is that it would somehow become less if told to others – welcome to my world of mental health! Yes, it is possible to take a story of faith, a really good story of faith, and make it vulnerable because it is the story of a vulnerable man. Over the last year I've determined to tell my story a little bit more. I even determined to make myself include it in a book. You see, I've come to realize that what I thought was 'my' story is actually God's story, and it is the story of all those young Christian men in a sixth form at a grammar school. It is the story of the teachers who faithfully enabled the Christian Union to meet, one of whom was the school woodwork (design technology) teacher, and it is the story of all those amazing people who listened as I started to talk about what had happened. Nearly 30 years ago, when I eventually told the Christian boys about what had happened, their joy truly surprised me. Now I understand their joy. It was the joy of heaven at one who was lost being found by the Saviour who so loves us that he seeks us out.

Our stories are his gift to his Church. They are to be shared and held to support us through times of great trial, when our troubles overwhelm us, when life is no longer worth living. I'm learning how to share my story so that I might equip my friends who are faithful: equip them with the story to tell me, of the faithfulness of the Saviour who seeks us out, who sought me out; a story that will remind me of who I am in Christ when I don't know who I am in myself. I know those times of despair; I know they will come around again and again until I meet my Saviour face to face and, once and for all, all pain is gone.

Our stories of Jesus, of being found in him, are our stories of confidence and assurance, our stories of faith. Share them with your friends, let them know who you are, equip them for the day when they need to sing those songs of faithful love over you as they sit by the fireside in the lament of your despair. Faith is confidence in what we hope for and assurance of what we do not see. Sometimes we need those who journey with us to hold that confidence and assurance for us. We need to trust their faithfulness as they enable our faith in the one who is ever faithful.

8

Hope

There was a particularly frustrating young woman when I was at university. I'd entered as a 'mature student' at the grand age of 22. Having been told I wasn't clever enough to go to university when I was 18, it was a complete surprise when, exploring ordination in the Church of England, someone said to me, 'We think you've got a brain, you should go to university and explore it.' I'd been working with people with learning disabilities since leaving school, and the decision to go to university was a surprise to everyone, including me. It was amazing to enter an environment with lots of 18-year-olds who had no idea how to cook or wash their clothes. Having been fully 'trained' in all things domestic as one of two men on the staff team of a residential home, it turned out I was a helpful presence in the university launderette, advising on wash type! It was also amazing to encounter young people with a sense of inner confidence, something that was unfamiliar to me, as my inner confidence was so 'inner' I'd never found it. The frustrating young woman was one of the 'inner confidence' people. She was a member of the Christian Union, and one day she came up to me and said, 'Rob, why do you walk around with your head looking to the ground?'

I stopped and pondered her question, thinking that looking at where I was going was perfectly sensible if I didn't want to trip over. But before I could come up with a pithy answer, she followed up her question with a statement: 'You're a child of the King. You should walk with your head held high!'

I can't remember what my reply was. I think it was a mumbled, 'Er . . . yes, hmmm . . . right, good point . . .', combined with a healthy dose of profound embarrassment. Lift my head up! A child of the King! Who on earth did she think she was, uttering such senseless, pride-fuelled rubbish! You can probably tell I didn't take it well – not that I ever let on. Replaying that scene 25 years later, I know now what my reaction was: pain. Inside, those words of encouragement and hope entered a deep wound of shame, and I was afraid that the King didn't actually love me. I was angry about the pain that she caused me and, anyway, despair had done its usual brilliant task of sucking all hope out of me. How could I lift my head to the horizon? What would I see? Would I see the one who made himself known to me in a vision, a presence, a piercing light? I wasn't brave enough to look.

It is sometimes said that there are two types of people in the world: people who, when they see a glass half filled with water, see it either as half full or half empty. I'd like to add a third category, because I'm married to someone who not only sees the glass as half full, but overflowing, bursting, such is her level of optimism. My wife, however, would want to add a fourth category of person. You see, I'm a *There is no glass* person. I don't see it as half empty, I see the disaster of what little water there is running away with nothing to hold it or protect it. You'd think we'd cancel each other out, but we don't. The combination of my post-traumatic stress disorder and long-term mental health means that I'm hyper-vigilant. I'm hyper-vigilant to the unfolding disaster that is continually about to happen before me, which makes hope rather tricky to see or imagine. However, the upside of hyper-vigilance is that I'm never knowingly under-packed and my wife knows that everything (*everything*) we need will always be in the suitcase for a holiday.

But according to the writer of the letter to the Hebrews, we have a promise that God has made, a promise God swore by himself, a promise that God has fulfilled in Jesus, who has entered the inner sanctuary, behind the curtain: 'We have this hope as an anchor for the soul, firm and secure' (Hebrews 6.19a). Jesus is our anchor of hope. He is the fulfilment of the Father's love, firm and secure for all eternity; nothing in all creation can separate us from his extra-ordinary love. For a man who cannot see the half-full glass, knowing there is hope that despair can never overcome, never suck dry, is vital. Like the sun above us, hope in Jesus, our anchor of hope, is constant, vital, life-giving, warming to the very soul, and always present regardless of whether or not we can see it.

That image of the hope of Christ like the constancy of the sun above is one I first heard at a conference, and it has stayed with me ever since. A Spanish psychologist, who was speaking at a major Christian conference, described his flight from Spain to the UK. It had been a wet and windy day when his plane took off from Madrid Airport. Clouds covered the sky and everything was dull; there was no sunshine to be seen or felt. He described the plane taking off, buffeted by wind and rain as it climbed up into the clouds where all vision was lost; the only thing he could see from the plane's windows was grey cotton wool of rain clouds. It was then that it happened. He described how suddenly the plane left the enveloping hold of the clouds and burst into the sunshine. As the plane climbed higher to reach its cruising altitude, the vivid blue sky became clear and the sun shone brightly. And then he realized: the sun had been shining all along. The storm clouds that had covered his view of the sun were temporary, but the sun's warmth and radiance were permanent, constant, ever present. And so he encouraged us never to lose hope of the constant love of Jesus, because he is always present, always loving, always constant. The storm clouds of life may blow across, blocking our vision, buffeting our lives, but the Son of God is still radiant.

Time and again, as depression and anxiety have blown across, blocking my ability to see or feel the warmth of Jesus, I have reminded myself to trust in the truth that he is still there, he is our anchor of hope, the clouds will pass, they always do, and I will see his glory once more.

Psalm 40 is my favourite psalm, particularly the opening two verses:

I waited patiently for the LORD;
   he turned to me and heard my cry.
He lifted me out of the slimy pit,
   out of the mud and mire;
he set my feet on a rock
   and gave me a firm place to stand.
(Psalm 40.1–2)

I love the description of the pit as 'slimy', containing 'mud and mire'; it's a miserable pit, which you can't get out of on your own. The whole of the psalm is born of a conflicted mind, wrestling with reality and hope. But the slimy pit; well, I don't know if you've ever tried to get out of a slimy pit. It's impossible to get a foothold; you dig your fingers into the side and the slimy mud just comes away in your hand. You exhaust yourself trying and trying to haul yourself out, forever sliding back to the bottom, ever more tired, ever more despairing that there is no way out. That pit has become the best description I have of living with a long-term mental health condition. 'Pull yourself up!' cry the people from outside of the pit. 'Come on, keep going, you can do it!' 'Pull yourself together!' 'Don't give up!' All the while standing there like Job's companions, in the warmth of the sun, proffering their 'advice' while you're the one doing all the hard work and gradually feeling, ever more hopelessly, with every slimy slip back to the bottom of the pit, that you can't do it yourself.

Oh, I know that slimy pit well. Even now I can see the dark miry mud, the marks in the walls of the pit where my fingers have been dragged back down by the weight of my despair. Time and time again I have wrestled the pit and lost. Lost back into its lonely muddy bottom to sit alone, staring at my pitiful existence and the impossibility of escape. It was in one of my many slimy pit moments that I suddenly remembered the echo of a voice from years ago. The Lord in his grace reminded me of a young woman who once said, 'Lift up your head . . .'. Did you know that when you're sitting in a slimy, miry, muddy pit with no way out, if you look up you can see the sky? It's there above your head. All the time you've been struggling, wrestling, despairing, the bright light of day has been present. The pit doesn't have a roof; there is nothing to block the daylight, only the forgetfulness of despair.

It was in that slimy pit moment, as I was reminded to look up, that I also remembered the verse and a half of Psalm 40 before the slimy pit:

> I waited patiently for the LORD;
>> he turned to me and heard my cry.
> He lifted me out . . .

You see, the only way out of a miry pit is through the hand of another. You can shout down all the advice you like, it won't make a bit of difference to the person in the pit. You can try and scramble your way out, but all the pit will do is consume you. What those of us in the pit need is the hand of another, the hand of the one who rescues us. I have found this to be a powerful call to hope and a powerful call to patience.

In the slimy pit, hope is the action of waiting patiently for the one who has come and is coming. Hope is not a desperate expense of energy. Hope is not the advice of another. Hope is the Lord and his everlasting goodness. Hope is knowing the one who turns to us and hears our cry. Hope is knowing that the Lord God Almighty has done this in every generation over thousands of years, and this hope is enacted in patient waiting. Now, it's not nice waiting at the bottom of a slimy pit. It's a miserable place. I'm grateful for the therapy and medication that has helped me in that place of waiting. I'm grateful for my amazing wife and close friends, who have the courage to come and sit in the pit with me, keeping me company, singing the songs of the Lord, reminding me of the vast horizon above.

Reading the psalms, an important discovery for me was the 'pivot of hope'. You will find the pivot of hope in many of the psalms. It is when the psalmist is in full flow of desperation and throws in a 'but' or 'yet'. That 'but' or 'yet' is the pivot away from despair to hope. 'My enemies outnumber me, yet . . .', 'Despair overwhelms, but . . .'. The pivot of hope has become my moment of taking a long deep breath when I'm in the miry pit. It causes me to pivot my head upwards, to change my perspective – yes, I am overwhelmed by troubles without number, but those troubles without number can never overwhelm the goodness of God. God is God, God reveals himself, the Father has revealed himself in the Son in the power of the Spirit. My overwhelming troubles cannot change that fact because I am not God, thanks be to God!

When I was younger, in my first counselling sessions with the man who chose my case, one of the most helpful questions he asked me to reflect on when my paranoia was in full flight during one counselling session was, 'Are you telling me that you are a mind reader?' It was a question that pulled me up short at the time. I wanted to yell back at him, 'Yes I'm a flamin' mind reader. I can read what people are doing. I can see what they're going to do to me . . .', but I didn't because I realized it wasn't true; I couldn't read other people's minds, I couldn't read his. It turned out I could barely read my own. The pivot of hope is that moment. That moment of pause, when the world stops, when everything is put on hold, and for a dazzling moment hope is seen.

The practice of the pivot of hope has become vital to me. It is a hopefulness I've sought to nurture when my feet are back on solid ground once more, set firm upon the rock of our salvation, Jesus Christ. I've discovered that God does indeed put a new song of praise in my mouth, a song of hope. There have been times when I've spent years in the slimy pit. Sometimes the pit lasts months, sometimes only days, but practising hope when not in the pit has slowly equipped me with the patience to wait when all that surrounds me are the dank, dark, miry walls once more. I have learnt to practise the pivot of hope and cry out to the Lord, patiently waiting in the secure hope that he is coming.

Alongside the pivot of hope, when I'm out of the pit I also practise what I describe as 'the naivety of hope'. This naivety of hope is the commitment to hope even when hope looks foolish or lacking wisdom. It means giving people the benefit of the doubt. It means imagining that what looks impossible could be made possible. It means imagining a world, or even a church, where people do love one another with a love that is utterly Christ-given. I've been called out for this in meetings. On one occasion I dared to imagine that a group of organizations could work together for the sake of the gospel. Another participant pointed out the folly of my hope as this had never been achieved before. I explained that I wouldn't surrender the naivety of hope because it was hope for the sake of the gospel of Christ.

The naivety of hope is open to disappointment, it takes the rough with the smooth, it knows that people are broken and sinful and will let you down. The naivety of hope tells you that when you're sitting in the pit, help is on the way, even when you can't see it, hear it or feel it. Perhaps key in this for me has been that my practice of the naivety of hope has taught me to see the glass of water, with a profound thankfulness that it is simply there and will be there. It has taught me to live as a disciple of the kingdom that has come and is coming, to see beyond what is and see what will be – I am pivoting, a naive hope-filled man, longing for my Saviour to come.

It isn't that in my pivoting naivety I've forgotten my journey so far – I haven't. I still know the effect of trauma, of abuse, of fear, shame, anger, despair. I haven't escaped from them; I won't, not until I see my Saviour face to face, because I live in a world that is broken, corrupted by sin and shame. The only way I could avoid them would be to lock myself away and refuse to engage with anyone anywhere in some crazed survivalist way, waiting for the day of my death, or the Lord, to come! No, my journey is about his hope. Without the journey I have travelled I wouldn't know Jesus and I wouldn't know that hope has won, in the most beautiful act of love: 'God demonstrates his own love for us in this: while we were still sinners, Christ died for us' (Romans 5.8). Neither would I know that my suffering has produced perseverance, perseverance has produced character, and character has produced hope. 'And hope does not put us to shame, because God's love has been poured into our hearts through the Holy Spirit, who has been given to us' (Romans 5.5). Hah! Take that, despair, and clear off back to your corner once again – hope does not put us to shame! Hear that? Hope does not put us to shame! I could dance! Oh shame, oh shame, where is your sting! I wonder, my friend, would you remind me of that when next I sit in the slimy pit?

If you have a friend in the slimy pit, hold out hope for your friend, because they may not be able to hold it for themselves. Save your advice, your 'wise words' and turn them into prayer. Pray, sing and share with them the psalms in which hope pivots and causes us to look up and see the sky above. I quite like it when I'm sitting in the pit and someone wanders along and, instead of telling me what to do, simply looks up to the sky and wonders at its beauty, its warmth, its sunshine. It causes me to stop and look and see. And if you're in the slimy pit, then welcome; it turns out there's a lot of us who know it well. It's a flippin' foul place to be; but – wow! The sunshine above, that blue sky, reminds me of another time, another place that I know will one day return. It reminds me of firm ground beneath my feet, a solid rock that holds me up. Look up and see the hand of the one who has come and will come again, and know the hope of divine love that has never and will never disappoint.

9

Love

I've always found the apostle Peter to be a compelling figure in the story of Jesus, although I'm fairly sure that had I been part of the group of women and men following Jesus two thousand years ago, I would have been the 'harrumphing disciple' standing back with his arms folded, finding Peter's passion, zeal and impulsiveness outwardly infuriating but inwardly inspiring. Peter, who went on to have a role of great importance in the very earliest days of the Church, had left his nets to follow Jesus and, in his passion to follow Jesus, walked on the water he once fished.

Peter is complex, as shown by his interaction with Jesus in Matthew 14 after the miraculous feeding of the five thousand. Caught up in a strong wind, the boat was buffeted and rocked by wind and waves, a situation that would not have been unfamiliar to Peter. The unfamiliarity came as he looked out and saw Jesus walking across the water towards the boat of disciples. 'Lord, if it's you,' – the conditionality present in Peter's voice – 'tell me to come to you on the water.' Seriously! 'Tell me to come to you'? This 'harrumphing disciple' would have been sitting in the boat hoping that Peter would sink in the waves of his own stupidity.

I know where my 'harrumph' comes from – it is rooted in my desire to have the same freedom as Peter to respond to the love encountered in Jesus.

We know the rest of the story, it's there for us to read. Jesus tells Peter to come to him. Peter gets out of the boat, starts walking, gets distracted by the wind, fear grips him, and he begins to sink. I wonder if the disciple John, who was later to reflect in a letter, 'but perfect love drives out all fear', ever held Peter in mind as he reflected on that night-time encounter between love incarnate and human fear. That encounter is the reality of our state and the challenge of love.

When my eyes are not fixed upon Jesus, the one who loves me and has called me to follow him, I begin to sink. I sink into the swelling sea of my ego that longs to be the sole object of my desire. I sink into the fear of my shame that would swallow me up into the shadows that exist in deep places. My sinking is not a metaphorical experience, it is utterly physically consuming, and it has an impact on the lives of those closest to me. Yet when I yield to love, when I fix my gaze once more upon Jesus, then the water becomes as solid as love incarnate. To walk upon the water is to walk upon love. The love of Jesus is as physical and evident as his incarnate self. He is the fullness of the Father's love, utterly sufficient, and in him I am fully loved.

I have been privileged to visit two amazing places: the Holy Land and Rome.

Standing on the shore of the Sea of Galilee, I have found myself wondering if I would have had the same crazy courage as Peter, the naivety of hope to step out of the boat on to, and not into, the water.

Standing next to Peter's tomb under St Peter's Basilica in Rome, I have pondered if I would have had the courage to make Peter's journey of discipleship, from the open horizon of the Sea of Galilee to the imperial might of Rome, the splendour of the Forum, the terror of the Circus and ultimately death. In the middle of the square outside St Peter's is an ancient Egyptian obelisk. It is placed there as it is thought to be the last thing Peter saw before he died, martyred for the one he loved. It is a reminder to those who wield power in the Church that their power is temporal and not eternal. Yet what was the first and the last thing that Peter saw? It was Jesus Christ, love eternal, the one who had called him to follow and the one upon whom Peter had fixed his gaze, his heart captured by the relentless love of the one who surrendered all that is seen and unseen for him, for us.

I love Jesus, but my love is like the butterfly ever attracted to the next sweet thing, distracted by the colour of the new, blown about on the wind of my own desires. How I long simply to fix my gaze upon him. To look upon him and be utterly lost in wonder, for I have been found in his love.

As I've grown older and have understood more the impact of trauma on my brain, I've slowly come to appreciate the grace in my butterfly-like state. My inability to focus at times, and the ease with which I'm distracted, are merely symptoms of my past played out in my present. I used to worry that I was failing as a Christian, that my inability to be consistent in my love, to be attentive and focused, was a sign of my utterly pathetic excuse for Christian discipleship. However, it turns out that the driving out of fear by perfect love is the journey of a lifetime, and some days fear has the upper hand.

'God is love', the apostle proclaimed at the end of a sentence that started 'Whoever does not love does not know

God' (1 John 4.8). I love people. I love my wife. I loved the people I served when I worked for Mencap Homes Foundation. I have loved the people I've served in parishes. I love my friends. I'm working really hard on loving my enemies. I love God. I love Jesus. I love the Father, Son and Holy Spirit. I'm not perfect. I've not got it all right, I'm not consistent, but I love my life, I adore Jesus for who he is and the wondrous grace he has poured into my life.

But every time, and I do mean every time, I'm floored by the commandment that he gave: 'Love your neighbour as yourself.' Dear Lord, if you wanted to give a gut punch, that was the one; asking me to love my neighbour as I love myself. I have no problem with the 'neighbour' bit; well, not much of a problem – it depends on the neighbour. But '. . . as I love myself'! Crikey! Lord, do you have any idea how ridiculous that sounds? I don't love myself. In fact, it isn't that I don't love myself, because that is a statement without the power of what I've actually felt in my life. I loathe myself. I loathe my very existence. I have in my mind the echo of years that tell me what a pathetic excuse for human existence I am. How in all that is seen and unseen could I possibly love that which is me? Yet Jesus loves me: this I know, and cannot deny.

Trauma weaponizes love. It turns what should be beautiful and inspiring into something that is torturous and painful. It took years for me to be able to acknowledge that my wife loves me. In the earlier years of our marriage, whenever she said 'I love you', my response would be something along the lines of 'You don't have to', 'I don't know how you can', 'I don't understand what that means', and yet within me a deep well of love existed for her. And here is the great divine wrestling match for all those of us who live with trauma, with long-term mental health conditions: the love of God has been poured into our hearts by the Holy Spirit. Love exists within us, divine love resides in our innermost being, whether we want it there or not. And that love, that divine love, is passionate about us and is transforming us from the inside out, whether we realize it or want it, because the activity of God in creation is not dependent on our permission. 'Not dependent on our permission' is a powerful and painful realization for a survivor of abuse. Getting a grip on 'permission' as an adult has been a point of safety for me through which I've been able to secure my safety. The realization that God's love is not dependent on my 'permission' is both wonderful and threatening at the same time.

There is a passage in Scripture that I return to time and time again. I can't find an answer to it. I've tried; I've tried to construct an interpretation that would allow me to exist in my perfect world of loving God, loving others, and yet excluding myself from love entirely. However, every time I've tried to apply my construct it has wilted in the fierce light of divine passion. Paul wrote:

> For I am convinced that neither death nor life, neither angels nor demons, neither the present nor the future, nor any powers, neither height nor depth, nor anything else in all creation, will be able to separate us from the love of God that is in Christ Jesus our Lord.
> (Romans 8.38–39)

It turns out my self-hatred is unable to separate me from the love of God that is in Christ Jesus our Lord. It's not listed there, but Paul adds this annoying catch-all, 'nor anything else in all creation', which means I have no get-out clause whatsoever.

For a long time, I understood that Jesus' call to love my neighbour as myself was dependent upon my ability to demonstrate love towards myself first, that somehow I had to draw upon the empty wells of wondrous love I felt for myself and offer that non-existent love to another. I thought I was an utter failure as a Christian, which also fitted neatly into my self-loathing (nothing like a little self-reinforcement to keep the fires of self-hatred burning brightly). However, this had been a fundamental misunderstanding on my part. I thought that the ability to love was dependent upon my non-existent resources, but it isn't. I love because he first loved me. I love because the eternal love of heaven has been poured out into all creation. I don't have to love with my love, but with that love that the Father through the Son has already poured out by the Spirit within me, because in Christ Jesus I am a new creation. I have entered a new status of relationship.

I explained in an earlier chapter that I'm unable to have children, and the way that had exposed another part of the reality of shame in my life. I don't have birth children; however, I do have two adoptive sons. Very early in our marriage my wife and I spoke about a shared call to adopt and a desire to see this expressed as we grew older together, sharing our life with someone else. We never realized at the time that adoption would be the means through which our sons would enter our lives. Adoption is joy birthed in tragedy. The trauma of the removal of children from a birth family or parent is a deep and lasting wound. However, in the UK, adoption is a means of seeking to give children in profoundly complex situations renewed hope. Our sons have both a birth family and a for-ever family. In our lives we work to weave the story of the two together: they are our and another family's sons. Our privilege is to journey through this part of their lives with them. For me, adoption has been a deeply profound lesson in love.

My sons are remarkable. We were gradually matched with them as we were assessed regarding our suitability as potential adoptive parents. We received their details months before we met them. We knew their story, met foster carers, teachers, social workers, psychologists – the list seemed endless. Our sons knew that a for-ever family were being sought for them, but they only knew about my wife and me 24 hours before they met us for the first time. Our sons are courageous and resilient. Having a seven-year-old and a five-year-old move in was a life-altering experience, though 'life-altering' is too tame a description – universe-changing seems closer to the truth. The fact that they were somehow able to trust to the extent that they were prepared to move in with us still causes me utter amazement.

My sons are remarkable teachers. They have taught me how utterly self-orientated my life was before they arrived, and daily teach me about how love is rich, deep and power-ful. I'd thought that in my journey of Christian disciple-ship I had learnt something about how to think of the other person, how to give of myself; it turns out I had no idea. The pain of our first months as a new family took many forms, but for me it was the pain of discovering the reality of my selfishness; that I had shaped my life around thinking about me, and my wife (though you may have already noticed in this story that thinking of my wife is not my major life skill), and that shaping life to two boys was going to be very, very challenging. I came face to face with the realization of my error in understanding the nature of love. As I struggled with my non-existent resources to love, I had to confront the limitations of my understanding.

Paul writes in Romans 8 about our adoption as children into the family of God and that, through adoption, 'The Spirit himself testifies with our spirit that we are God's children' (Romans 8.16). Paul's use of adoption is contextual; his audience understood that adoption in Roman society meant being given the full legal standing of an heir. It is remarkable that God so loved us that he has reshaped creation itself by stepping into our lives in Christ Jesus, that our adoption is his initiative, his extravagant love, his desire to enter the profundity of our trauma of separation, and renew relationship through himself.

In love I enter my sons' experience of trauma. This is my initiative. I cannot simply sit back and wait for them; love compels me to enter into the reality of their lives and make love known to them and for them. For a man who has struggled to feel love and acknowledge love, this has been a fundamental change in my life for which I am deeply thankful. I had no idea of the love that the Father held for us. If the passionate, compelling love I feel for my adoptive sons is so all-consuming, then how extravagant is our Father in heaven's love?

This love that dwells within us, which is the Spirit at work, is a love I cannot deny. I can't say it isn't present, because it enables me to love and love my sons even when they drive me crazy. That love is a love I am slowly learning; it is the love that I offer to my neighbour, because it is the love that I know for myself, the love of the heavenly Father for his child. It is the love made passionately known in Jesus, and this wonderful reliance upon the ever-reliable love of Jesus brings the most glorious freedom: the freedom to love another with the same divine love that we are loved with. And it is a freedom, because I cannot lock it away, I cannot inhibit this love because it does not submit to fear. I am able to love myself as my neighbour with the same love that Christ has given me. The wonder of this love is like the warmth of the sunshine above. It is never-failing.

My mental health will fail again. I will end up in my slimy, miry pit once more. I will feel utterly loveless and unlovable. But I cannot deny the love of God in Christ Jesus; to do so would be to lie to myself, and many years ago after meeting Jesus I promised that I wouldn't become the liar I had accused others of being.

The gradual realization of this heavenly love has been wonderful for me, but what about those around me and closest to me? They are the ones who hold the greater calling, to hold out the gift of love to one who rejects their love, who considers himself to be unlovable. Well, I am slowly learning to be thankful for them. It is a slow journey of learning, because it means acknowledging that my feeling of being unloved and unlovable is unreliable, and even untrue. For the reality is that the love that those close to me hold out for me and to me is the reality of love incarnate. If you are someone who is in relationship with a person who lives with the effect of trauma and mental health, thank you for being someone who loves and loves and loves. Thank you for offering the reality of love eternal in Christ Jesus, for it is only love eternal that can fill a void of love that seems to last for ever.

As a father, I long for my sons to be filled up with love, yet I know the reality of our lives is that this will be a lifelong journey. I am thankful that our heavenly Father has shown us such grace in the Son; that the reality of our lives is that we will be one day filled up with love, the day we are welcomed home and we behold our Saviour face to face. Until that time we are filled daily with the Father's love through the activity of the Spirit, because each day we leak a little, each day we drop our heads a little, each day we can feel empty, and each day we need to be reminded afresh that the hope of God is love incarnate: Jesus Christ. And ultimately, the love of Jesus is all sufficient. Hallelujah!

Conclusion: Setting sail

I still enjoy sailing. I enjoy sailing a small dinghy on a lake, gradually making my way across from one point to another. That's the thing when you sail on a lake: you sail from one point to another. You note what your point of sailing is – it might be a buoy or an object on the shore, and you sail towards that point. The challenge comes as you make your way towards your point. The wind may change direction or strength, affected by the landscape that you pass by. It is remarkable how the shape of a hill or a woodland can suddenly cause a steady constant breeze to stop, or swirl around in its direction, disorientating you from your point of sailing. You look back to check where you've come from, you look ahead to find your point, and you adjust your course and sail accordingly to maintain direction. It's hard work responding to the changes, moving your body, adjusting sails, all to maintain forward momentum.

When Paul set off on the journey that would take him under arrest from Caesarea to Rome via three different boats, I wonder what he thought his point of sailing was? What was the point, the marker, he was heading towards? This question about Paul's journey struck me as I was sailing across a lake heading towards a large white buoy on the surface of the water. There I was, heading towards the buoy, which was my immediate point of sailing, but what was my long-term marker? What was the point to which I was travelling in my journey of life?

Under house arrest in Rome, Paul reflected on his life, considering all that was behind him and his passion to know Christ and the power of his resurrection. He wrote: 'Not that I have already obtained all this, or have already arrived at my goal, but I press on to take hold of that for which Christ Jesus took hold of me' (Philippians 3.12). Paul's point of journey was Jesus. It was Jesus who had called him, and Jesus he was travelling to. Yes, he was battered and buffeted, he had to change direction on more than one occasion, adjust his sail and set his face towards his point of sailing once more, but his vision wasn't simply what was immediately before him, it was set upon Jesus and his journey home to the heavenly realm.

This is our call: to fix our sight upon Jesus and press on towards him. It is the call of all of us who follow after Jesus, having left behind the immediacy of our lives to begin an adventure that will lead us heavenwards – this journey will never look perfect, but it can look obedient – obedient in our longing to acknowledge our fear, to speak honestly about our shame, to dig deep as we dispel the roots of anger, and in despair to acknowledge the gifts that surround us even in our pain. And in all of this, to surrender to Jesus, for he surrenders all for us, and in surrender know that faith, hope and love are never absent. They are close at hand. The storms may blow across our horizon but the warmth of the Son is ever constant.

So I've set my course. I will be rocked, buffeted, knocked off course; I will have to adjust my sails, replace parts that fail. I know this because it is part of my life. But this I know also: the one who calls us is faithful and our journey home is to him – Jesus Christ, our Lord and our Saviour.

Notes

1 K. Golding and D. Hughes, *Creating Loving Attachments: Parenting with PACE to nurture confidence and security in the troubled child* (London: Jessica Kingsley, 2012).
2 W. Brueggemann, *The Message of the Psalms: A theological commentary* (Minneapolis, MN: Augsburg Press, 1984), p. 76.

WE HAVE A VISION OF A WORLD IN WHICH EVERYONE IS TRANSFORMED BY CHRISTIAN KNOWLEDGE

As well as being an award-winning publisher, SPCK is the oldest Anglican mission agency in the world.

Our mission is to lead the way in creating books and resources that help everyone to make sense of faith.

Will you partner with us to put good books into the hands of prisoners, great assemblies in front of schoolchildren and reach out to people who have not yet been touched by the Christian faith?

To donate, please visit www.spckpublishing.co.uk/donate or call our friendly fundraising team on 020 7592 3900.